PHILLY'S FIT-STEP®
WALKING DIET

LOSE 15 LBS., SHAPE UP, & LOOK YOUNGER IN 21 DAYS

FRED A. STUTMAN, M.D.

MEDICAL MANOR BOOKS
PHILADELPHIA, PA

Medical Manor Books are available at special quantity discounts for sales promotions, premiums, fund raising or educational use. Book excerpts can also be created to fit special needs.

For details write the
Special Markets Dept. of Medical Manor Books
3501 Newberry Road, Philadelphia, PA 19154

Phone: 800-DIETING (343-8464)
E-mail: info@medicalmanorbooks.com
Website: www.medicalmanorbooks.com

OTHER BOOKS BY THE AUTHOR:

Walk, Don't Run. Philadelphia: Medical Manor Press, 1979.

The Doctor's Walking Book. New York: Ballantine Books, 1980.

The Doctor's Walking Diet. Philadelphia: Medical Manor Books, 1982.

DietWalk: The Doctor's Fast 3-Day SuperDiet. Philadelphia: Medical Manor Books, 1983. Pocket Books® Edition, Simon & Schuster, New York, 1987.

Walk, Don't Die. Philadelphia: Medical Manor Books, 1986. Bart Books Edition: New York, 1988.

Walk To Win: The Easy 4-Day Diet & Fitness Plan. Philadelphia: Medical Manor Books, 1990.

Diet-Step: 20/20-For Women Only. Philadelphia: Medical Manor Books, 2001.

Diet-Step: For Seniors. Philadelphia: Medical Manor Books, 2003.

100 Best Weight-Loss Tips. Philadelphia: Medical Manor Books, 2005.

100 Weight-Loss Tips That Really Work. New York: McGraw Hill Books, 2007.

Dr. Walk's Power Diet-Step. Philadelphia: Medical Manor Books, 2009.

The Case of the Unwanted Pounds. Philadelphia: Medical Manor Books, 2011.

Philly's Fit-Step® Walking Diet
Lose 15 Lbs., Shape Up, & Look Younger in 21 Days

Publisher's Cataloging-in-Publication
(Provided by Quality Books, Inc.)

Stutman, Fred A.
Philly's fit-step walking diet: lose 15lbs., shape
up & look younger in 21 days / by Fred A. Stutman, M.D.
—First edition.
pages cm
Includes bibliographical references and index.
LCCN 2013913973
ISBN 978-0-934232-34-0
ISBN 978-0-934232-35-7

1. Fitness walking. 2. Reducing exercises.
3. Physical fitness. I. Title.

RA781.65.S78 2014 613.7'176
QBI13-600184

First Edition 2014
Manufactured in the United States of America

To:

Suzanne

Robert, Mary, Samantha, Alana

Roni, Paul, Geoffrey, Eddie

Craig, Christine, Rain, India

& Sparkey

ACKNOWLEDGEMENTS

EDITOR: Suzanne Stutman, Ph.D.

CONTRIBUTING EDITOR: Craig M. Stutman, Ph.D.

TEXT EDITOR: Geoffrey A. Bruskin

PERMISSIONS: The American Academy of Family Practice; J & J Snack Foods, Inc.; The Physicians' Health Bulletin; Dr. Walk's Diet & Fitness Newsletter

WORD PROCESSING: Accu-Med Transcription Service

ILLUSTRATIONS: Steve Oswald, Norm Rockwell, Judit Meszaros

COVER DESIGN: Steve Oswald

TEXT DESIGN: Erin Howarth

PUBLISHER: Medical Manor Books, Philadelphia, PA

FIT-STEP® is the registered trademark of Dr. Stutman's Fitness Walking Program.

DIET-STEP® is the registered trademark of Dr. Stutman's Weight-Loss Program.

DR. WALK® is the registered trademark of Dr. Stutman's Diet & Fitness Newsletter. REG. U.S. PAT. OFF.

DIETWALK® is the registered trademark of Dr. Stutman's Quick Weight-Loss Plan.

CONTENTS

AUTHOR'S CAUTION

IT IS ESSENTIAL THAT YOU
CONSULT YOUR OWN PHYSICIAN
BEFORE BEGINNING THE PHILLY
FIT-STEP® WALKING DIET.

-Fred A. Stutman, M.D.

INTRODUCTION

I originally formulated this weight-loss, fitness, and body-shaping plan for my patients in Philadelphia, who like most of you wanted a healthy, easy, and effective way to lose weight and get fit quickly. By following this diet and fitness plan, you will be able to boost your energy level, lose weight, and build muscle in only 21 days. You will feel better, look younger, and actually live longer on the Philly Fit-Step Walking Diet. The weight you lose will stay lost forever and the fitness you gain will last you a lifetime. At last, a diet and exercise plan that really works and keeps on working. I've developed this Diet & Fitness Plan for my patients and readers, by combining a healthy diet plan with an aerobic walking program and easy strength-training exercises. This easy-to-follow plan will help you lose weight quickly, re-shape your body, and boost your energy and fitness level. You will lose weight, shape up, and look younger in just 21 days.

There are no severe restrictions of any particular food group, except for foods that are high in saturated fats. This truly unique quick weight-loss plan is formulated exclusively for those individuals who are tired of unhealthy, low-carbohydrate fad diets. The diet is very easy to follow, and there are no special meals to prepare or complicated recipes to follow. The diet works just as well in a restaurant as it does at home. And I'll actually show you how to eat a Philly Cheesesteak that's low in fat and calories.

Philly's Fit-Step Walking Diet combines a healthy low-fat, high-fiber, lean protein diet with an aerobic walking program and easy-strength training exercises. The body-shaping component does not involve strenuous exercises, lifting heavy weights, or working out on weight machines at the gym. This unique combination of aerobic and strength training exercises deliver a double-blast of calorie burning for complete cardiovascular fitness, permanent weight-loss, and complete body-shaping. This plan will show you how to lose weight permanently, feel and look younger, and live longer. And, believe it or not, you can actually lose up to 15 pounds and 3 inches in only 21 days.

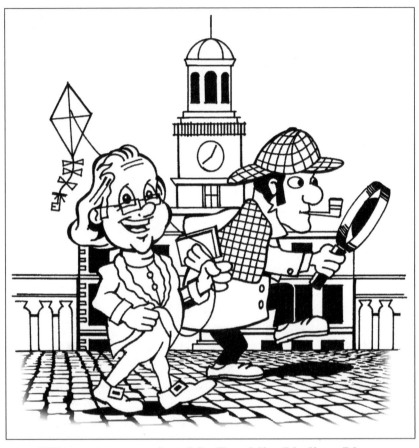

"Elementary, my dear Mr. Franklin. I believe I have solved the mystery of why a good many of the citizens of Philadelphia are overweight: They never walk!"

1

PHILLY'S 40/40 FIT-STEP® DIET

As a family practice physician in Philadelphia and having written numerous books and medical articles on diet, nutrition and exercise, I've figured it was about time to write a book about a unique, medically formulated diet and exercise program that I've developed for my Philadelphia patients over many years of medical practice. A good percentage of my patients have benefited immensely from this diet and fitness plan which is called the Philly Fit-Step Walking Diet. This plan consists of an easy-to-follow healthy diet, and an aerobic exercise walking program, combined with easy strength training exercises.

I'd like to share the success stories of my Philadelphia patients with the rest of the country's overweight and under-exercised individuals, whom I'm sure could benefit from this healthful diet and exercise plan. The Philly Fit-Step Walking Diet will give everyone the opportunity to participate in a successful and permanent weight loss and fitness plan. The plan is designed for busy people who don't have a lot of time or energy to follow complicated diet plans or strenuous exercises. At last, an easy weight loss, fitness, and body shaping plan for anyone, regardless of body size or fitness level. This easy-to-use plan will work for you whether you live in Philadelphia or San Francisco.

The Philly Fit-Step Walking Diet combines a unique, medically formulated weight loss plan, which limits your total saturated fat intake, and increases your intake of high-fiber, lean protein foods, along with healthy monounsaturated fatty acids. This diet provides all of your body's necessary nutrients and limits your fat intake for good health. By combining a diet low in saturated fat with moderate lean protein and high fiber foods, in combination with an aerobic walking plan, you will be able to lose weight quickly and permanently while developing cardiovascular fitness. On the Philly Fit-Step Walking Diet, you also get the added benefit of living a longer, healthier life, since this plan provides protection against many of the diseases of aging, such as heart disease, high blood pressure, stokes, and many different forms of cancer. Here's a unique diet and exercise plan that helps you lose weight while looking younger and living longer.

UNHEALTHY FAD DIETS
SHERLOCK HOLMES & THE PHILADELPHIA CONNECTION

In the late 19th century London, it took the famous detective Sherlock Holmes to unmask a den of nefarious diet-scam scoundrels and thieves from the depths of London's seamier side. The notorious and devious organizer of these diet scams was a certain Professor James Moriarity, who was not only a brilliant mathematician, but was also known as "The Napoleon of Crime." He was found to be formulating a variation of the bogus low carbohydrate diet for the unsuspecting, obese upper class in London's posh neighborhoods. Moriarity created a spider's web of diet scam thieves throughout all of London. These scoundrels fleeced the well-to-do Londoners out of their pounds, by selling them a bill-of-goods on the so-called weight-loss benefits of these dangerous low carbohydrate diets. These obese people were only too happy to consume mass quantities of beef, mutton, game, and cheese along with their beer and wine.

It took all of the deductive and reasoning powers of Sherlock Holmes to convince these unfortunate, rotund individuals that they were putting their health and in fact, their very lives at considerable risk. He informed them that the weight that they initially lost on this low carbohydrate diet was in fact only water weight, and he further confirmed that the weight that they did lose would come back tenfold once they stopped the diet...provided they didn't die first. Many a wealthy Londoner went to an early grave before Holmes was able to put a stop to this nefarious scheme. As Sherlock Holmes once said to Dr. Watson, "It is an old maxim of mine that when you have excluded the impossible, whatever remains, however improbable, must be the truth." In a singular adventure, which remains unpublished to this date, John H. Watson, M.D., chronicled these events in a little known monograph entitled, *The Case of the Nefarious Diet-Scoundrels.*

Once Sherlock Holmes finally unmasked this dangerous low carbohydrate diet program, these devious diet scoundrels along with Professor Moriarity quickly fled from London, and it is thought that most of them set-sail for America, where their descendants still reside. Many of these descendants are thought to have taken up residence in our nation's birthplace, the city of Philadelphia. These diet-scam descendants artists began again, in an attempt to convince the American public of the so-called weight-loss benefits of these dangerous low carbohydrate diets. Unfortunately, like the unsuspecting Londoners, many Americans were putting their health, as well as their lives at risk by following these unhealthy diets. Fortunately, the first American women's magazine, *The Ladies Home Journal,* which was published in Philadelphia in 1883, exposed these diet charlatans to the American public. This article was published in part due to the efforts of Benjamin Franklin, whose healthy eating motto for the good people of Philadelphia was, *"Eat to live, not live to eat."* Philadelphians were also encouraged to walk more frequently for their health, in part due to the way that William Penn, the founder of the Province of Pennsylvania, laid out the streets in the city of Philadelphia in a grid-like pattern. These easy to follow street patterns, made walking around in all of the different areas of Philadelphia a more pleasant experience.

After the publication of this article in *The Ladies Home Journal,* and due to the efforts of Benjamin Franklin, these nefarious scoundrels quickly disappeared from sight. They resurfaced again in America in the mid 1900s with a variety of new books and pamphlets again touting the so-called benefits of these low-carbohydrate fad diets. It was recently discovered that a direct descendant of Sherlock Holmes, known only as Dr. Walk from the city of Philadelphia, helped to unmask these diet charlatans as being completely untruthful. Not unlike Benjamin Franklin, who was a proponent of healthy eating habits, Dr. Walk informed the American public about the hazards of these unhealthy diets and about the benefits of a truly healthy diet. He also showed the people of Philadelphia how they could improve their health and fitness just by walking the streets of Philadelphia. This information has been herein set forth in this new monograph, entitled *Philly's Fit-Step Walking Diet.*

MODERN DAY DIET CHARLATANS

So, how do people actually lose weight on all of those low-carbohydrate, high-fat diets? For example, they say you can have bacon and eggs for breakfast, a hamburger for lunch, and a juicy steak for dinner. Sounds tempting, doesn't it? They also tell you that you can't have any, or at the very least, limited amounts of carbohydrates with each meal. For instance - no vegetables, fruits, cereals, breads, potatoes, pasta, or any whole-grain nutritious foods. Sounds unappetizing and unhealthy, doesn't it? It certainly is! And yet, over 75% of the commercially available diet books and diet plans work on this abnormal metabolic process principle.

The simple fact is that you do lose weight initially on these very low carbohydrate, high fat, high protein diets; however, most of the initial weight loss is water weight loss due to a metabolic process called *ketosis*, a condition found in unhealthy patients (for example: those people with diabetes and kidney disease). Once the body gets rid of the water, it starts burning leftover fat—which, in itself, is a good thing; however, the downside is that this abnormal process of ketosis also begins to burn the body's protein (muscle tissue). This is a very bad thing. By attempting to burn protein as a source of fuel for energy, the body is actually breaking down one of its most important elements, since protein is used to sustain life (building and repairing the body's tissues, cells and organs). In such a scenario, a substance called ketones will appear in your urine (a by-product of this abnormal process called ketosis), giving you clear evidence that your body is breaking down its muscle tissue. This is one of the reasons that fatigue and general weakness have been reported as early side effects of this completely unhealthy diet. Also, kidney and liver damage may result if too much of the body's protein is broken down from these unhealthy low carbohydrate, high protein, and high fat diets. To make matters worse, these diets are deficient in vitamins, minerals and essential nutrients.

These rapid weight loss programs (low carbohydrate, high fat, and high protein diets) also have the added downside of what is called "rebound weight gain." This occurs after the initial water weight loss, which is followed by the breakdown of fat and protein used for energy production (fuel). The body's carbohydrate stores then become depleted because of the very low intake of carbohydrates in these diets, and thus, there is a limited availability of carbohydrates to be burned as a fuel. Actually, carbohydrates are designed to be the very first type of calories burned as fuel in our normal metabolic process.

Once your body becomes aware that it is carbohydrate depleted by exhibiting the symptoms of fatigue, malaise, muscle cramps, and decreased urine output (occurring after the initial water loss), then your brain's control center receives stress (SOS) signals from all of the body's cells suffering from carbohydrate depletion. Once your brain's central control center receives this flood of distress messages, it immediately realizes the need for a cheaper source of fuel (refined carbohydrate and sugar) to prevent brain damage from the lack of glucose that the brain needs in order to function. Just when you're feeling exhausted and fatigued by this low-carb diet, your hunger center sets you off on a carbohydrate binge, to counteract this lethargy you've been feeling for weeks or months. At this point your body begins to accumulate fat deposits, hence the term "rebound weight gain." Eventually, your sweet tooth is satisfied, and you attempt to resume your unhealthy diet of excess fat and low carbohydrates. Not a healthy situation by any means.

SAY GOODBYE TO UNHEALTHY DIETS

Most people realize that the so-called "ideal weights" found in health magazines are completely unobtainable. One of the main problems with dieting is the fact that people who are on diets binge-eat far more often than non-dieters. Dieters do not eat according to whether they feel hungry, but actually out of the false notion that they are being good or bad. If in fact they eat a dessert that they feel "is bad for them," then frustration and anxiety set in and they take new oaths to do better the next time.

When you start limiting your food intake, neurochemicals in the brain respond as if the body is starving itself. The metabolic rate slows down so that the body does not burn food as quickly in order to survive, which the body actually perceives as starvation. This calorie deprivation produces food cravings, which are the opposite effect of what you are trying to achieve. The psychological and physiological effects of dieting can therefore be devastating. In our culture it is very easy to dislike our bodies. The mirror becomes the enemy, and we feel captured in our reflections. It is only natural that we aspire to be released from the prison in the mirror.

According to behavioral psychologists, children left to themselves will select a variety of foods, and will stop eating when they have had enough. Adults on the other hand, will identify foods as either being good (healthy) or bad (unhealthy), and on this basis attempt to make their selections. The road to normal eating is to stop listening to the myriad of advice concerning what to eat, and to start following your own biological and physiological needs for essential healthy nutrients. Snacking on junk food occasionally is fine, and as long as you do not beat yourself up over it, you will survive nicely. On the other hand, if snacks are restricted permanently, then your brain's neurochemical transmitters will send you into a binge-eating frenzy. Once your brain is satisfied with an occasional small self-satisfying snack (such as a piece of fruit), your brain's appetite control mechanism (appestat) will keep your hunger under control for longer periods of time, and will let you concentrate on a diet that's really healthful.

SAY HELLO TO PHILLY'S BEST WALKING DIET

Remember, you live in your body and you do not have to make drastic changes in order to feel good about yourself. *Philly's Fit-Step Walking Diet* will enable you to lose as much weight as you want to in order to feel comfortable with your body. You will also develop maximum cardiovascular fitness, a firm, toned body and boundless energy on this wonderful new program. This plan was developed for my patients, who like most of you, were tired of the endless, short-lived fad diets and the myriad of strenuous exercise programs that were completely unrealistic.

The problem with most diet and exercise programs is that they are too complicated. There are too many tables to consult, too many diet meal plans to prepare and too many strenuous exercise programs to follow. Most of these plans don't consider that everyone has a life to lead that is packed full of a hundred things to do each week. People don't really have the time to follow complicated or time-consuming diet or exercise plans. The beauty of Philly's Fit-Step Walking Diet is that it is designed especially for women and men who have limited amounts of time for diet and exercise, but who, on the other hand, would like a simple, easy, effective weight-loss and fitness plan that doesn't interfere with the rest of their lives. It's that simple! It doesn't take a lot of your valuable time, and it actually works!

I originally developed this program for my patients in Philadelphia, who, like most of you, wanted a diet and exercise plan that doesn't interfere with day-to-day living. You'll be delighted at how easy the program is, and how well it works. The Philly Fit-Step Walking Diet is easy to follow and will help you to lose weight, keep fit, and stay healthy. There are no complicated diet plans to follow, nor any weight-loss clinics to join. Also, there is no need to join a gym or engage in any strenuous exercises. This is an easy to follow, effective weight-loss program and fitness plan with a minimum of time and effort on your part. Also, this weight-loss program is geared towards your individual body build, and your own metabolic rate. This combination plan of a healthy diet and an aerobic walking plan will also boost your energy level and keep you fit, as you burn off unwanted fat calories.

PHILLY'S FIT-STEP® WALKING DIET

STEP 1: DIET-STEP® 40/40 PLAN

The first step consists of a diet of no more than 40 grams of total fat and no less than 40 grams of fiber each day. This quick weight-loss formula combines foods that are low in saturated fats and high in heart-healthy monounsaturated fats. Also, the diet limits unhealthy refined carbohydrates and substitutes healthy, high fiber, complex carbohydrates, consisting of fruits, vegetables, nuts, seeds, beans, and whole-grain products. This quick weight-loss diet also adds healthy lean protein for energy, fitness, and appetite control. The Diet-Step: 40/40 Plan lets you lose weight at your own pace without complicated diet plans, counting calories, fad diets or starvation techniques. The plan is relatively easy and quite effective for losing weight quickly and maintaining the weight that you've lost.

The Diet-Step plan is the first medically formulated quick weight-loss formula for people of all ages and body builds. No matter whether you're slightly overweight or obese, short or tall, athletic or unconditioned, young or old, muscular or flabby—this is the perfect weight-loss plan for you. All you have to do is **limit your total fat intake to no more than 40 grams daily (concentrate on heart-healthy, monounsaturated fats) and eat at least 40 grams of high fiber foods every day.**

This unique diet is a healthful, life-long diet plan for weight loss, weight control, and good health. As you will see in the following chapters, the plan is easy, inexpensive, safe, effective, and works quickly to help you lose weight, achieve maximum physical fitness, and develop a shapelier figure. It will keep you in excellent health for the rest of your life.

1. Eat no more than 40 Grams of Total Fat Daily (concentrate on heart-healthy monounsaturated fats with omega-3 fatty acids), such as olive, canola, and peanut oils; nuts and seeds, avocados, olives, fish,and flax seed). Severely limit intake of saturated fats, particularly red meat, to a maximum of 20 grams daily.

2. Eat no less than 40 Grams of High Fiber Complex Carbohydrate foods daily, consisting of fruits, vegetables, nuts, beans, lentils, chickpeas, seeds, and whole-grain foods.

3. Eliminate refined bad carbohydrate foods (sugar, white flour, white rice, and white pasta); processed and packaged foods; baked goods (pastries, biscuits, cookies, crackers, etc. made with trans-fats: hydrogenated or partially hydrogenated oils).

4. Eat moderate amounts of lean protein foods, consisting of fish, white poultry meat, lean lamb and veal, low-fat dairy foods (milk, egg whites, cheese, yogurt, tofu, and soy) and vegetable protein products (avocados, soy, nuts, beans, and lentils) and whole grain products.

5. Fruits and vegetables are allowed in almost unlimited quantities.

6. Limit the amount of salt, caffeine, and alcohol in your diet.

7. Drink at least six 8 oz. glasses of water daily.

STEP 2: FIT-STEP® WALKING: 40 MINUTE PLAN

This second step consists of 40 minutes of an aerobic exercise walking program six days per week, for an additional calorie burning power boost. Walking also produces a fresh supply of oxygen surging through your blood vessels to all of your body's tissues and cells. The Fit-Step Plan boosts the weight-loss power of the Diet-Step Plan by burning additional calories with a 40 minute aerobic exercise walking plan six days per week. Or you can divide your walk into two 20 minute walks daily. On the Fit-Step plan you will also develop maximum cardiovascular physical fitness, good health, and longevity.

STEP 3: FIT-STEP BODY-SHAPING PLAN

The third step is the body-shaping plan which includes both the **Diet-Step Plan** and the **Fit-Step Walking Plan.** The Body-Shaping plan also adds **weight-bearing, strength-training exercises** to your walking program, which in effect produce a double-blast of calorie burning, by combining your 40 minute aerobic exercise walking program with strength training exercises. Strength-training also strengthens and builds your muscles and bones, and boosts your metabolic rate so that you continue to burn calories long after you stop your exercise. This is easily accomplished by using light-weight, hand-held weights during your 40 minute walk three days per week, or you can divide your walk into two 20 minutes sessions daily. This plan, in addition to helping you lose weight, will actually sculpt and mold all of your body's muscles and give you a shapelier figure. There is no need to do strenuous exercises or power weight lifting in order to get perfect body-shaping. This diet and exercise walking program will help you to lose weight more quickly by burning additional calories.

PHILLY'S BEST DIET & FITNESS TIPS

1. **Decrease the amount of saturated fats** in your diet (fatty meats, fatty fowl like duck and dark meat of chicken and turkey, whole dairy products including butter, margarine, and hydrogenated or partially hydrogenated oils (corn, palm, safflower, and other vegetable oils). These oils are present in the form of trans-fats contained in prepared, packaged and processed foods like chips, cookies, crackers, cake mixes, frozen dinners, margarine, vegetable spreads and any and all products that contain trans-fats. Limit your total fat intake to no more than 40 grams daily for good health and weight-loss. By limiting your total fat intake, you will automatically limit your intake of unhealthy saturated fats. Remember to concentrate on the heart-healthy monounsaturated fats.

2. **Increase the amounts of heart-healthy monounsaturated fats** in your Philly Fit Step Walking Diet plan. Concentrate on olive, canola oils, and peanut oils, nuts and seeds, all types of beans and legumes, avocados, and egg whites. Use non-fat milk, yogurt and cheeses and soy protein products. Also include the new heart healthy, trans fat-free vegetable spreads. These spreads contain healthy monounsaturated fats and heart-healthy omega-3 fatty acids, like olive oil.

3. **Concentrate on high fiber, complex carbohydrates foods** with a low glycemic index to prevent spikes in insulin levels, which cause sudden drops in blood sugar and results in fat being deposited in your fat cells. Concentrate on eating healthy whole grain breads, cereals, pasta, and other whole grains such as bran, wheat germ, bulgur, quinoa, and whole grain noodles and rice. Increase your intake of fruits and vegetables, avocados, sweet potatoes, nuts, seeds, beans and legumes. Consume at least 40 or more grams of fiber daily for good health and weight-loss. Fruits and vegetables are allowed in almost unlimited quantities. This high-fiber diet component of the Philly Fit-Step Walking Diet is a life-long diet plan for weight loss, weight control, good health and longevity.

4. **Eliminate refined, so-called bad carbohydrates from your diet.** These include all white processed grains, pastas, breads, rice, corn and white potatoes. Eliminate all refined sugar and white flour products. Stay away from packaged foods and processed products (cakes, pies, candies, crackers, cookies and most desserts), except for fruits, since they all contain high amounts of refined sugars. Refined sugar causes your blood sugar and insulin levels to peak, which in turn increases your appetite and stores unwanted fat deposits in your body.

5. **Consume healthy lean protein fats**. Add healthy vegetable protein, such as nonfat milk, low fat cheeses including yogurt, soy proteins like tofu, and egg whites. Also include beans, nuts, beans, legumes and whole-grain products. It is also important to add some animal protein to your diet, especially fish, and also white meat of poultry without the skin, and very limited amounts of lean cuts of lamb, pork and beef (small portions only with all of the fat trimmed off).

When you are on a low calorie diet, your body needs more protein for the production of energy and your body's cell maintenance. Protein is the essential nutrient responsible for the maintenance and repair of all your organs, tissues, muscles, bones, and brain cells. All foods are sources of energy; however, protein provides a greater boost in energy levels since it is absorbed slowly and thus produces a constant source of energy.

6. **Stay away from harmful protein.** Most high protein diets have you eating 3-4 times more protein than the recommended dietary allowance, and in most cases, the high protein you are actually eating is the harmful, high saturated kind of fat. These diets tax your kidneys and leach out calcium from your bones, in addition to contributing to elevated blood cholesterol, heart disease and strokes. Minimize harmful protein like fatty meats, fatty poultry with the skin intact and whole dairy products such as whole milk and dairy products, butter, vegetable oils (except olive, canola and peanut oils), and egg yolks. However, egg yolks have gotten a lot of bad press over the years, and recent research has shown that 4 or 5 egg yolks per week can actually be beneficial because of their high content of protein, nutrients, and antioxidants. Even though they are high in cholesterol, they are extremely low in saturated fat.

7. **Limit the amount of salt, caffeine and alcohol** in your diet. Excess amounts of salt and caffeine in your diet can raise your blood pressure and excess caffeine may cause heart rhythm abnormalities. Both salt and caffeine can actually increase your appetite. Excessive alcohol intake can add unwanted calories to your diet (7 calories per gram) and could possibly damage your liver over time. However, 4 ounces of red wine daily can be heart-healthy, since it contains a powerful antioxidant called *resveratrol*.

8. **Drink at least six 8 oz. glasses of water daily.** Water fills you up so that your appetite is decreased, especially if you drink 8 oz. of water before your meals. Also, water is necessary for all of your body's metabolic functions to work properly, including maintaining the electrolytes in your blood at a proper balance. An adequate amount of water in your diet also contributes to proper kidney function. If you're not hydrated properly you can develop palpitations, headaches, dizziness, weakness, heat exhaustion, and eventually dehydration. Very severe dehydration can thicken your

blood cells and could possibly lead to convulsions, heart attacks and strokes.

9. **Walk 40 minutes six days per week for fitness and good health.** You can divide your daily walk into two 20 minute sessions, if that's more convenient for you. Walking is the very best and safest aerobic exercise. Walking regularly helps your body deliver a steady supply of oxygen to all of your body's cells, tissues and organs. This increased blood supply of oxygen to your body's cells keeps your body's metabolism in perfect balance and helps you to burn extra fat calories so that you can lose weight quickly and safely. Strenuous exercises can do considerably more harm than good.

10. **Also, walk for 40 minutes (or two 20 minutes sessions) using light-weight, hand-held weights, three days per week**, for maximum calorie burning, weight-loss, fitness and body-shaping. This addition of weight-bearing exercises adds strength-training, muscle-building and additional calorie burning to the walking-exercise workout. These strength-training exercises will shape your body's muscles, which leads to a trimmer, shapelier figure. This double-blast of calorie burning from the aerobic effects of walking, combined with the additional calorie-burning from the strength-training exercise, is what makes *Philly's Fit-Step Walking Diet* the very best diet and fitness plan ever developed.

SIMPLE STEPS TO EFFECTIVE WEIGHT LOSS

1. **Eat several small meals a day.** It's natural to be a little hungry during the first few days of the diet; however, a diet that leaves you hungry all of the time will eventually lead to overeating. Hunger is just a physical sensation and you can easily overcome it. Most people find that eating anywhere from four to six meals per day works best for alleviating hunger.

2. **Don't deprive yourself of treats.** If you deprive yourself of treats for any length of time while you're on a diet you'll end up binge-eating at some time during the diet. Add a treat, such

as a small piece of dark chocolate, or a low-fat low calorie fruit protein bar, or a piece of fruit. Also, a great snack is a fresh fruit smoothie with low-fat yogurt prepared in your blender. Give yourself this type of treat at least every-other-day. These added calories won't affect your diet at all.

3. **Clean out your cabinets and cupboards.** Throw away all of those high fat, high sugar goodies and snack foods (chips, cookies, cakes, etc.) that prove tempting when you're hungry or fatigued. Also divide large bags of snacks (nuts, raisins, rice cakes, whole grain cereal, etc.) into single portion plastic baggies. Or, as an alternate, buy 100 calorie low-fat, pre-packaged snacks.

4. **Keep a food journal.** For the first four weeks of your diet, write down everything you eat, so that you can estimate the total number of calories and grams of fat that you eat daily. If you find that the total calories or grams of fat are above what you thought would be good for your diet, then adjust your diet the next day. Don't weigh yourself every day. It's not necessary to weigh yourself more often than once a week. If you weigh yourself every day, you will get frustrated and eat more.

5. **Let everyone know you're on a diet.** Tell your family and friends that you would appreciate their support, since losing weight is important to you. People who eat meals with you should be cognizant of the fact that they shouldn't try to influence you as to what to eat, or offer you a taste of their meal. It's also important to choose food wisely, especially when eating in a restaurant, and not be influenced to order foods that your dining companions are eating.

6. **Start a regular walking exercise program for 40 minutes every day.** Walking not only burns calories, but it also boosts your metabolism and builds muscles, especially when you combine walking with strength training exercises. See walking with handheld weights in Chapter 10. An interesting way to keep track of your walking program is to buy a pedometer.

7. **Change your life, not your diet.** There are many short-lived, fad diets; however, if you want to be healthy and lose weight, then you'll have to develop good eating and exercise habits, and remember that weight loss and fitness are gradual processes. There are no fast or immediate results. Rome wasn't built in a day, and neither were you. If you change your life-style insofar as eating healthy and exercising regularly, then the weight loss and fitness results that ensue will be easy to achieve and long lasting.

8. **Stay motivated.** By concentrating on what you as an individual can accomplish by staying fit, feeling strong and healthy, you will be more inclined to stay motivated. It's easy to occasionally skip a day or two of your exercise program or your diet plan. It's ok, if you don't beat yourself up over it. Just get back on track and stay motivated by keeping your eye on your goal of good health, weight loss and fitness. These rewards will come all in good time, and will last you a lifetime. Remember, a healthy diet and exercise program will add years to your life, and life to your years.

9. **Eat only when you're hungry.** Most people eat for emotional reasons, like when they're stressed or anxious. Compulsive eating is a disorder that's difficult to break, but once broken, it is easy to prevent from reoccurring. The key is to eat only when you're hungry.

10. **Have an apple or two a day.** Having a couple of apples between meals every day will fill you up without filling you out. In fact, people who snack on apples between meals consume fewer calories at mealtime, and are considerably less likely to become obese. And apples of course contain healthful nutrients.

11. **Schedule your snacks for mid-afternoon.** Plan your snacks the night before. Have a mini box of raisins or one-quarter cup of mixed nuts, or a small bowl of oatmeal with cinnamon, or a piece of fruit.

12. **Keep low-fat, lean protein meals on hand.** A can of tuna packed in water makes a tasty snack using low fat or non-fat mayo on a whole wheat muffin or whole wheat slice of toast.

- A slice of low fat cheese on one slice of whole wheat toast with non-fat mayo or mustard.

- Skinless chicken breasts can be cooked in advance and stored in the freezer, and then when needed defrosted in a microwave and stir-fry with veggies or add low or non-fat mayo and make a quick chicken salad (with celery or cucumber) on a bed of lettuce.

13. **Eliminate the whites.** Refined white flour, white rice or sugars are made up of empty calories, without any nutritious value. Whole grain foods, on the other hand, are chock-full of nutrients, vitamins, minerals and fiber, and these foods satisfy your appetite control mechanism quickly, even when small amounts are eaten. However, when you consume white flour, sugar, white rice, and other processed foods, you will develop quick spikes in blood sugar, which leave you feeling hungrier. Most processed foods also contain excess amounts of sodium, which can cause elevated blood pressure and lead to weight gain by retaining fluids.

14. **Don't be afraid of all fats.** Heart-healthy omega 3 fatty acids are found in fatty fish (salmon, tuna, halibut and haddock), flax seed, soybeans, avocados, olives, and seeds and nuts. These are healthy sources of monounsaturated fats.

15. **Don't skip breakfast.** People who miss breakfast often consume significantly more calories during the day, especially mid-morning. A healthy, low fat breakfast with high fiber and moderate protein, such as an egg-white omelet with veggies, or a small bowl of whole grain cereal with fruit and skim milk, will keep your hunger at bay all morning long.

The Philly Fit-Step Walking Diet is a healthy balanced diet and walking program comprised primarily of:
- 40 percent healthy, complex carbohydrates made up of fruits, vegetables and whole grained products, including legumes, beans, soy and flax seed.

- 30 percent heart-healthy fats, such as olive and canola oils, nuts (almonds and walnuts), fatty fish, and avocados.
- 30 percent protein—fish, white meat of chicken without the skin, very lean cuts of meat, egg whites and non-fat dairy (milk, yogurt, tofu and soy products), nuts, seeds, beans, and whole grain products.

Walk 40 minutes six days per week or 20 minutes twice daily. Walk with light-weight, hand-held weights for 40 minutes or 20 minutes twice daily, three days per week.

Philly's Fit-Step® Walking Diet combines a healthy low-fat, high-fiber, lean protein diet with an aerobic walking program and easy-strength training exercises. On this plan you will boost your energy level, lose weight, and develop permanent cardiovascular fitness. Your body will become thinner, your muscles and bones stronger and your figure firmer and shapelier. This plan will show you how to lose weight quickly, get fit, shape up, and feel and look younger. You can actually lose up to 15 pounds and 3 inches in only 21 days.

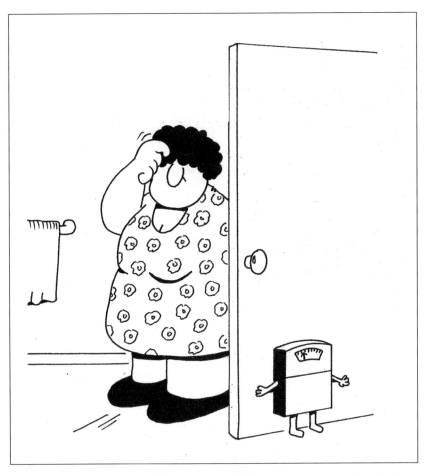

"Maybe she won't see me. My springs won't take another diet again."

2

LOSE 15 LBS. IN ONLY 21 DAYS!

Diet-Step®: 40 Grams of Fat and 40 Grams of Fiber is a quick and easy weight loss plan. No doubt about it! It is the only medically formulated diet plan that really works and keeps on working. Weight loss is fast and easy, and what's more—it's permanent. There is no rebound weight gain, no food cravings, no starvation techniques, no liquid protein drinks and no diet pills. There are no unhealthy low-carb diets to follow, where you end up stuffing your face with meat, eggs, cheese, butter, cream, bacon, fat and more fat, until you and your arteries are ready to explode.

By limiting the total grams of fat to 40 grams daily, we eliminate many high fat calories that add extra weight and can block your arteries with saturated fat and cholesterol. Remember that each gram of fat contains 9 calories compared to 4 calories from each gram of protein and carbohydrates. It's quite easy to calculate that eating a gram of fat adds considerably more weight to your body than eating a gram of protein or carbohydrate. The high fiber content (40 grams per day) in this diet also provides a built-in mechanism against gaining weight by regulating your appetite control mechanism known as the *Appestat*. Fiber fills you up without filling you out. This is because in addition to being low in calories, fiber has a high water and bulk content which satisfies your appetite quickly.

The Philly Fit-Step® Walking Diet is specifically designed for people of all ages, all shapes, all sizes and all weights. The weight loss component of the Fit-Step Walking Diet is the Diet-Step® 40/40 plan which is easy to follow and works quickly to shed all of the extra unwanted pounds that you want to lose. This easy plan is essentially a diet that is high in fiber, complex carbohydrates and lean protein. This diet limits your intake of saturated fats, cholesterol, refined carbohydrates, sugars, salt, caffeine, and alcohol. When combined with a 40-minute walk or two 20-minute walks six days per week, your body burns additional calories to boost your metabolism. This plan has been shown to be effective in weight loss, weight control, fitness and good health. *You can actually lose up to 15 lbs and 3 inches in only 21 days by following the Philly Fit-Step Walking diet.*

QUICK WEIGHT LOSS ESSENTIALS

1. Eat no more than 40 Grams of Total Fat Daily (concentrate on heart-healthy fats and reduce saturated fats)

2. Eat no less than 40 Grams of Fiber daily.

3. Do not eat refined or processed foods (sugar, white flour, and white rice). Do not eat packaged or commercially baked goods made with hydrogenated or partially hydrogenated oils.

4. Limit salt, caffeine and alcohol.

5. Drink at least six 8 oz. glasses of water daily.

6. Walk 40 minutes or two 20 minute sessions, six days per week.

DIET-STEP®:40/40 MEAL PLANS

The basic diet is divided into easy to follow meal plans. These diet meal plans have already factored in 40 grams total fat/40 grams fiber per day without your having to add up the number of grams of fat and fiber. Once you've completed the first few weeks of your diet, these basic Diet-Step Meal Plans will become an automatic part of your everyday schedule. The diet is extremely easy to follow. There is no need to remember what to eat at home or what to order in a restaurant for any particular meal. Once you've become comfortable with the basic meal plans, you can then start to formulate your own individual meals by eating no more than 40 grams of total fat and no less than 40 grams of fiber daily. Consult the Fat and Fiber Counter in the Appendix, and then you can mix and match any individual meal that you'd like.

There is such a variety of foods included in this 40/40 diet that your taste buds will never tire of this healthful, nutritious, palatable diet program. By varying the foods in your diet, there are never any hunger pangs or food cravings. The Fat & Fiber Counter in the Appendix will allow you to choose any foods that you want. Remember, the Diet-Step plan is the only diet that in addition to controlling weight, will add years to your life by providing essential, healthful nutrients, antioxidants, phyto-nutrients, vitamins and minerals. These nutrients eliminate harmful free-radical components from your body. This is a diet and exercise plan for fitness and health as well as for weight loss and body-shaping.

After you have reached your ideal weight on this easy diet program, you will never again have to worry about rebound weight gain. The Diet-Step: 40/40 plan enables you to lose weight quickly and permanently, utilizing only these basic sample menu plans during your initial weight-loss program, or by following any of the optional meal plans that are listed at the end the basic weekly meal plans. Also, you can choose any combination of meals (breakfast, lunch and dinner) containing 40 grams of fat and 40 grams of fiber found in the Fat and Fiber Counter. *You are only limited by your own creativity.*

MONDAY

BREAKFAST	1 whole medium orange or ½ grapefruit ¾ cup cold whole grain or bran cereal with ½ cup any fresh fruit & ½ cup non-fat milk 1-2 cups coffee or tea (non-fat milk or 1% milk) 8 oz. glass water
LUNCH	1 cup soup (any type except cream based)—the more vegetables and beans, the better (e.g. minestrone soup) Use whole wheat bread to make a veggie sandwich with lettuce, tomatoes, sprouts, cucumber, carrots or any leafy green vegetable. Add Dijon mustard or small amount low fat mayo 8 oz. glass water
SNACK	Fresh fruit and low fat yogurt smoothie, or piece of fruit 8 oz. glass water
DINNER	4 oz. baked or broiled fish (scallops, shrimp, or any filet of fish) with 1 tsp. extra virgin olive oil, season with kosher salt, onion powder, and lemon pepper. Add lemon as needed. 1 cup steamed veggies (broccoli, cauliflower, etc.) and 1 small baked yam 1 whole-wheat dinner roll 4 oz. red wine or 12 oz. light beer 8 oz. glass water
SNACK	½ cup raisins or 6 pitted prunes, with 2 tbs. nuts (almonds, pecans or walnuts) *-or-* 1 cup mixed fresh fruit (strawberries, blueberries, blackberries purple grapes, bananas, etc.) 8 oz. glass water

Total grams fat: 39.8 Total grams fiber: 40.2
WALK 40 MINUTES DAILY

TUESDAY

BREAKFAST

Fried egg using PAM® on whole wheat English muffin with non-fat whipped butter-like spread. Add slice tomato and ½ slice low-fat cheese.
1 medium orange or ½ cup strawberries or ½ ruby grapefruit
1-2 cups coffee or tea (non-fat milk or 1% milk)
8 oz. glass water

LUNCH

1 slice pizza (tomato only or light cheese), topped with your choice of green peppers, mushrooms, onions, or garlic. Blot the pizza with a paper napkin several times to absorb excessive fat. No meat toppings.
1 large tossed salad with non-fat dressing
Drink of your choice (decaffeinated and sugar-free)
8 oz. glass water

SNACK

1 medium apple or any piece of fruit
8 oz. glass water

DINNER

4 oz. baked eggplant or zucchini casserole with marinara sauce and mozzarella cheese, baked in non-stick pan with Pam®. Lightly breaded with whole wheat bread crumbs dipped in egg whites
1 cup steamed veggies (cauliflower, broccoli, spinach, etc.)
1 slice whole wheat bread or roll
4 oz. tomato or low-salt vegetable juice
8 oz. glass water

SNACK

½ cantaloupe or melon with ½ cup blueberries, strawberries or raspberries *-or-* 1 piece of fresh fruit (banana, pear, apple, peach, plum, orange or nectarine) *-or-* ½ cup mixed nuts
8 oz. glass water

Total grams fat: 39.5 Total grams fiber: 39.0
WALK 40 MINUTES DAILY

	WEDNESDAY
BREAKFAST	1 whole medium orange *-or-* ½ small melon *-or-* ½ cup fresh fruit ¾ cup cold whole grain *-or-* bran cereal with ½ cup any fresh fruit & ½ cup non-fat milk 1-2 cups coffee or tea (1% milk or non-fat milk) 8 oz. glass water
LUNCH	1 cup soup (vegetable, tomato, lentil, bean, pea, celery, minestrone, consommé, chicken noodle/rice, Manhattan clam chowder—no creamed or pureed soups). ½ tuna fish sandwich on whole wheat bread with low fat mayo and lettuce and tomato 1 glass unsweetened iced tea 8 oz. glass water
SNACK	1 medium apple *-or-* ½ cup mixed raisins and nuts 8 oz. glass water
DINNER	Mozzarella, tomato, and basil salad with ½ tsp extra virgin olive oil 4 oz. whole-wheat pasta primavera (fresh veggies and ½ cup marinara sauce with or without mushrooms, garlic and small amount Parmesan cheese 1 whole wheat dinner roll 4oz. tomato or low-fat V8 Juice® 8 oz. glass water
SNACK	2 cups unbuttered, unsalted popcorn (hot air popcorn popper without oil) *-or-* 1 cup mixed fruits (berries, purple grapes, bananas) 8 oz. glass water
	Total grams of fat: 39.2 Total grams of fiber: 39.2 **WALK 40 MINUTES DAILY**

THURSDAY

BREAKFAST	6 medium dried or stewed prunes *-or-* ½ cantaloupe or honey-dew melon *-or-* 1 cup any fresh fruit 1 slice whole or cracked wheat bread (½ teaspoon whipped/diet oil-free margarine or 1 tsp. jelly) 1-2 cups coffee or tea (1% milk or non-fat milk) 8 oz. glass water
LUNCH	1 cup fresh fruit salad on bed of lettuce with ½ cup low-fat cottage cheese and 2 whole-wheat crackers *-or-* 1 small chef salad with turkey (2 slices) and low-fat cheese (1 slice) only; use lemon, vinegar or 1 tsp. non-fat dressing Diet drink of your choice (decaffeinated and sugar free) 8 oz. glass water
SNACK	Fresh fruit and low fat yogurt smoothie *-or-* piece of fruit 8 oz. glass water
DINNER	Large tossed salad (lettuce, tomato, celery, carrots, cucumber), with non-fat dressing 4 oz. broiled or baked chicken breast, skin removed; add seasoning (paprika, garlic, pepper, etc.) pan-sauteed in non-stick pan sprayed with Pam® or vegetable spray ½ cup brown long whole grain rice 1 cup steamed veggies (broccoli, spinach, or brussels sprouts) 4 oz. tomato or vegetable juice 8 oz. glass water
SNACK	⅛ slice angel food cake with non-fat whipped cream and sliced fruit or berries *-or-* 1 medium piece fresh fruit (apple, pear, peach, plum, banana, apricot or nectarine) *-or-* ½ cantaloupe or melon with ½ cup raspberries, strawberries or blueberries *-or-* ½ cup of raisins and mixed nuts 8 oz. glass water

Total grams fat: 39.4 Total grams fiber: 40.3
WALK 40 MINUTES DAILY

	FRIDAY
BREAKFAST	½ medium grapefruit 4 oz. (½ cup) fresh *-or-* unsweetened grapefruit juice ¾ cup cooked or cold whole grain (bran type) unsweetened cereal with ½ cup non-fat milk, ½ medium banana *-or-* 2 dozen raisins (½ oz.) *-or-* 6 pitted prunes 1-2 cups coffee or tea (non-fat milk or 1% milk) 8 oz. glass water
LUNCH	3 oz. (½ cup) tuna or chicken salad stuffed in whole-wheat pita bread (1 tsp. fat-free mayonnaise), with lettuce, tomato and cucumber. Use tuna packed in water. Diet drink of your choice (decaffeinated and sugar free) 8 oz. glass water
SNACK	1 medium peach *-or-* ½ cup mixed raisins and nuts 8 oz. glass water
DINNER	Large tossed salad with non-fat dressing (lettuce, tomato, celery, carrot, cucumber) 4 oz. baked or broiled fish (flounder, salmon, haddock, halibut, cod, sole, bass, bluefish, perch, trout) with lemon and 1 tsp. extra virgin olive oil 1 medium baked sweet potato or baked yam including skin (no butter, margarine or sour cream) 1 cup steamed vegetables (your choice) 4 oz. red wine or 12 oz. light beer 8 oz. glass water
SNACK	2 small unsalted, whole wheat pretzels or one medium soft pretzel (Superpretzel®) with or without mustard *-or-* ¾ cup non-fat yogurt or low-fat fruit cottage cheese with 2 tsp. wheat germ 8 oz. glass water
	Total grams of fat: 41.0 Total grams of fiber: 39.6 **WALK 40 MINUTES DAILY**

SATURDAY

BREAKFAST

2 eggs (one egg white) scrambled with tomato, green peppers, onions and any non-fat cheese *-or-* 1 poached or fried egg (non-fat, oil-free margarine – soft type)
One orange or tangerine or ½ melon or ½ ruby grapefruit
1 slice whole wheat, rye or pumpernickel bread with all fruit jam (1 T)
1- 2 cups coffee (non-fat milk or 1% milk)
8 oz. glass water

LUNCH

1 cup soup any type except creamed—the more veggies and beans the better
Large tossed salad with ½ tsp. olive oil & vinegar or non-fat dressing
2 whole-wheat crackers
Diet drink of your choice (decaffeinated and sugar-free)
8 oz. glass water

SNACK

Fresh fruit and low fat yogurt smoothie prepared in your blender

DINNER

3 oz. veal (lean) scaloppini or chicken (white meat without skin) cacciatore (baked with tomatoes, onions, peppers, mushrooms and garlic—your choice)
1 small baked or sweet potato with skin (no butter or sour cream)
1 slice whole wheat bread or roll
4 oz. tomato or vegetable juice
8 oz. glass water

SNACK

1 cup mixed fruit (berries, bananas, peach, grapes, kiwi, etc.) *-or-* 1 baked apple (artificial sweetener) and cinnamon and raisins *-or-* ½ cup frozen yogurt ice cream
8 oz. glass water

Total grams fat: 40.7 Total grams fiber: 39.7
WALK 40 MINUTES DAILY

	SUNDAY
BREAKFAST	2 small whole grain pancakes (e.g., buckwheat made with egg substitute or egg whites) topped with fresh fruit or sugar-free syrup One orange *-or-* tangerine *-or-* ½ melon *-or-* ½ grapefruit 1-2 cups coffee or tea (non-fat milk or 1% milk) 8 oz. glass water
LUNCH	Nicoise salad: tuna (dry), tomato, ½ sliced hard-boiled egg, (3) black olives, (1) anchovy, onion, bell pepper, radish and celery (balsamic vinaigrette dressing on the side—just a few fork-fulls) 1 glass unsweetened iced tea or lemonade 8 oz. glass water
SNACK	1 small box raisins *-or-* ½ cup grapes (purple or green) *-or-* 6 pitted prunes 8 oz. glass water
DINNER	3 oz. sirloin steak (lean) with grilled onions, mushrooms, garlic, peppers—your choice 1 medium baked potato *-or-* sweet potato with skin (no butter or sour cream) 1 cup steamed vegetables—your choice 4 oz. red wine or 12 oz. light beer 8 oz. glass water
SNACK	¾ cup sugar-free, fat-free ice cream *-or-* sugar-free Jell-O or pudding with non-fat whipped cream *-or-* ¼ cup mixed nuts (walnuts, almonds, cashews) 8 oz. glass water
	Total grams fat: 38.1 Total grams fiber: 41.2 **REST!**

OPTIONAL DIET-STEP® MEAL PLANS

The following lists are a variety of 40 Grams Fat/40 Grams Fiber options for your meal plans. Each meal (breakfast, lunch or dinner) has been pre-calculated to add up to approximately ⅓ of the allotted fat and fiber grams for any day. In other words, when you combine any 3 meals (breakfast, lunch & dinner), you'll have the total allotted 40 grams fat/40 grams fiber for any given day

DIET-STEP®: BREAKFAST OPTIONS

- 1 fried egg with non-fat spray and two small veggie non or low fat sausages made with tofu

- Egg white veggie omelet on a whole wheat English muffin

- 1 fried egg with non-fat spray and 1 slice whole wheat bread and 1 tsp. all-fruit jam

- 1 non or low fat waffle with fresh fruit topping

- Two small whole wheat or buckwheat pancakes made with egg whites or egg substitute topped with fresh fruit and/or sugar free syrup

- 1 poached egg with 1 slice whole wheat toast and 1 tsp. all-fruit jam

- ½ cup low-fat granola with ½ cup blueberries and strawberries and ½ cup skim or 1% milk

- 1 scooped-out whole wheat bagel with 1 slice unsalted smoked salmon (nova lox), with non-fat cream cheese, tomato, onion, lettuce, and capers

- 1 cup cold bran-type or whole wheat cereal with ½ cup any fresh fruit and ½ cup skim or 1% milk

- 2 egg whites or egg substitute omelet with 1 slice low-fat (skim milk) cheese, tomato, onions, green peppers, mushrooms (any or all)

- 1 cup cooked oatmeal or wheatena with cinnamon and ¼ cup raisins

- 1 cup fat-free yogurt with fresh fruit and 1 Tbs wheat germ

- 1 scrambled egg with non-fat spray and oat bran or whole wheat English muffin with 1 tsp. all-fruit jelly

- 1 toasted small whole wheat bagel with 1 tsp. non-fat cream cheese

- 1 slice cinnamon French toast with egg substitute and whole wheat bread

DIET-STEP®: LUNCH OPTIONS

- 1 whole-wheat bun with two slices reduced-fat turkey breast, with lettuce, tomato, mustard or 1 tsp non-fat mayonnaise

- 1 cup Chinese greens with 6 medium grilled shrimp with garlic, ginger, and scallions, with 1 cup brown rice

- 1 non fat or low fat cream cheese (2 Tbs) and jelly (2 Tbs) sandwich on whole wheat bread

- 1 whole-wheat bagel scooped out with 2 slices low-fat cheese, grilled with tomato and Dijon mustard or 1 tsp non-fat mayonnaise

- 1 whole wheat sandwich with two slices skim milk cheese (alpine lace) or other low-fat cheese, with lettuce, tomato, shredded carrots and sprouts, with mustard or 1 tsp. non-fat mayonnaise

- 1 small can vegetarian baked beans, 1 fat-free beef hot dog or fat-free turkey hot dog on whole wheat bun with sauerkraut, relish and mustard and small side salad with 1 tsp non-fat dressing

- 2 Tbs non or low fat cream cheese sandwich on whole wheat bread or whole wheat bagel with sprouts, tomato, cucumber, lettuce, and onions

- 1 medium whole wheat pita pocket with grilled chicken breast (3 oz) and 1 tsp. non-fat mayonnaise with lettuce, tomato, celery and cucumber

- Approximately 15 steamed mussels or clams with ½ cup marinara sauce, or in 1 Tbs white wine, 1 Tbs extra virgin olive oil with garlic, shallots, and parsley. Small side salad and whole wheat roll

- 1 Tbs reduced-fat peanut butter & 1 Tbs jelly sandwich on whole wheat bread

- 1 soft corn tortilla with ½ cup fat-free refried beans with shredded low-fat cheese, lettuce, tomato, salsa, and guacamole

- ½ veggie hoagie (tomatoes, lettuce, olives, peppers, onions, cucumbers, carrots, sprouts-your choice) with roll scooped out leaving only shell of Italian roll with 1 tsp low fat mayo or olive oil and oregano

- 1 medium whole wheat pita pocket with tuna (3 oz) packed in water with lettuce, tomato, cucumber, sprouts and 1 tsp. Dijon mustard or 1 tsp. non-fat mayonnaise

- 1 veggie burger on whole wheat bread or bun with lettuce, tomato, onion & ketchup

- 1 cup soup (minestrone, lentil, split pea or any vegetable or bean-based soup) with one small whole-wheat roll

- 1 can (3 oz) boneless and skinless sardines (drain oil) on whole wheat bread or pita with tomato, lettuce, onion, and Dijon mustard

- spinach salad with 1 oz low-fat blue cheese, ½ oz. chopped walnuts, sliced apples, cherry tomatoes, cucumbers, in 1 Tbs dressing made with mustard, lemon and 1 tsp olive oil

- panini sandwich toasted on scooped-out Italian or French roll with tomato, low-fat mozzarella cheese, basil and lettuce

- Nicoise salad with mixed greens, tuna, string beans, tomato, anchovies, ½ sliced hardboiled egg, olives, radishes, celery, onions and bell pepper with mustard vinaigrette dressing on the side (dip fork in dressing sparingly) and one scooped out French roll

- Goat cheese salad with reduced-fat goat cheese, mixed greens, tomato, olives, bell peppers, cucumber, celery, with mustard vinaigrette dressing on the side (dip fork in dressing sparingly) and one scooped-out French roll

- Open faced tuna melt on whole wheat bread with low fat Swiss or provolone cheese, with low fat mayo.

- Fruit and/or veggie smoothie prepared in a blender with low or non fat yogurt or 1% milk and soy protein powder

DIET-STEP®: DINNER OPTIONS

- 2 soft tacos with non-fat refried beans, lettuce, tomato, onion, grated non-fat cheese with 3 oz. sliced grilled chicken, salsa and guacamole

- 3 oz broiled or baked cod, halibut, mackerel or sole with grilled onions, peppers, mushrooms and tomatoes, with lemon, wine and seasonings, small whole wheat dinner roll and tossed salad with 1 tsp. low fat dressing

- 1 cup spinach fettuccine with fresh vegetables and ½ cup tomato or marinara sauce and large tossed salad with 1 tsp. low fat dressing

- Chicken Caesar salad with lettuce, tomato, chopped celery, cucumber and with 3 oz grilled chicken breast and non-fat parmesan cheese and 1 Tbs fat-free Caesar dressing

- 1 cup whole wheat spaghetti with 12 clams or mussels or 6 grilled shrimp, garlic, ⅓ cup white wine, 1 tsp olive oil and seasoning and large tossed salad with 1 tsp. low fat dressing

- 1 grilled 3 oz lean hamburger on whole wheat roll with lettuce, tomato, onion and ketchup and 1 small white potato made into oven-baked French fries (slice into fries, spray nonstick pan with non-fat spray and bake on 400 degrees until crisp)

- 1 small can of sardines (drain oil) or tuna packed in water in large tossed salad of lettuce or romaine, tomato, cucumber, pepper, onion, sprouts, carrots and olives and 1 tsp non-fat dressing or mustard-vinaigrette dressing

- 1 slice pizza (tomato, or with light cheese and tomato) topped with veggies of your choice and a side salad with 1 tsp non-fat dressing

- 3 oz lean roast beef with horseradish and small baked potato or yam with skin, 1 cup steamed veggies and small whole wheat roll

- 1 cup low-fat macaroni and cheese with 1 cup zucchini, diced tomatoes, onions and garlic and an ear of corn or a small sweet potato and steamed fresh carrots (½ cup)

- 6 medium cooked peeled shrimp with cocktail sauce and small ear of corn and 1 cup steamed asparagus, broccoli or spinach

- 4 oz. grilled salmon steak or salmon fillet with tomatoes, onions, peppers and garlic and small baked potato or yam and 1 cup steamed vegetable (your choice)

- 2 small lamb chops (trim fat) with 2 tsp. mint jelly and whole broiled tomato with 1 small baked sweet potato and tossed salad with 1 tsp. low fat dressing

DIET-STEP® NOTES

1. The above diets meal plans (breakfast, lunch and dinner) have been pre-calculated to contain no more than 40 grams of total fat and no less than 40 grams of fiber. To formulate your own combination of foods, just check the values in the **Fat & Fiber Counter** (APPENDIX) and mix and match any foods for any meals that you like. Remember to use no more than 40 grams of total fat and no less than 40 grams of fiber each day.

2. The most important part of the Diet-Step® Weight-Loss Plan is to keep the total fat content to no more than 40 grams daily and to concentrate on heart-healthy fats and limit saturated fats. Not only does this accelerate your weight loss, but you decrease your risk of heart attacks and strokes by reducing your blood cholesterol levels. By limiting your total fat to 40 grams daily and concentrating on the heart-healthy fats, you in effect limit your intake of saturated fats, dietary cholesterol and trans-fatty acids—all of which can significantly raise your blood cholesterol to dangerous levels. **According to the American Heart Association, for every 1% drop in blood cholesterol, your risk of a heart attack drops 2%. Pretty impressive!**

3. An equally important factor in this diet is the 40 grams of **dietary fiber** that you will be eating every day. Since fiber is primarily plant based, you will be eating lots of soluble and insoluble fiber (at least 40 grams), which also helps to reduce your cholesterol in addition to reducing your appetite. These high fiber plants also contain numerous beneficial compounds including phyto-nutrients, antioxidants, flavonoids, B & C vitamins, minerals, beta and other carotenoids, and folic acid, among others. All of these compounds help to fight heart disease, cancer and many other degenerative diseases of aging.

4. You will notice that it is not necessary to count and record the grams of cholesterol with each meal. They are listed in the Fat & Fiber Counter for your own information. The American Heart Association usually recommends no more than **300 mg. per day of dietary cholesterol**. However, by limiting your total fat intake to 40 grams/day, you will be automatically limiting your total intake of cholesterol. There are a few exceptions that we'll discuss later; for example, shell fish (shrimp, lobster and crab) which is high in cholesterol, but is not high in total grams of fat. Other fatty fishes like salmon, tuna, mackerel, herring, sardines and pompano, contain high amounts of **omega-3 fatty acids** which can significantly reduce your risk of heart disease. These omega-3 fatty acids are known as the heart-healthy fats.

5. Other **heart-healthy fats** include seeds, nuts, avocados, olives, and certain oils (ex. olive, peanut and canola oils). While these foods have a high total fat content, they are very low in saturated fats. They are also high in **monounsaturated fats**, which have been proven to be heart-protective. These foods can actually help to lower blood cholesterol and thereby reduce your risk of heart attacks. Nuts and seeds also contain many important vitamins and minerals, for example, selenium, which has been proven to be a potent cancer fighter. However, even these good fats have to be limited to some extent on the weight loss diet, since you can't exceed 40 grams of total fat daily. You will, however, be able to add more of these good heart-healthy fats to your diet on the maintenance diet plan.

6. It's the **saturated fats** that you have to concentrate on eliminating from your diet, so that you'll have more room for the heart-healthy monounsaturated good fats. You will also notice a column in the Fat & Fiber Counter (Appendix) marked "Saturated Fats." These are the dietary fats that come from animal sources. These saturated fats are dangerous and can block the arteries in your heart, brain and legs. This blockage

can lead to heart attacks, strokes and vascular disease. The American Heart Association recommends limiting saturated fats to no more than 15-20 grams daily. However, it is not necessary to count the grams of saturated fat on the Diet-Step® Plan. By limiting the total grams of fat to 40 grams daily, your intake of saturated fats will be far below the recommended values. Limit meat (beef, pork, veal) intake to no more than two small servings (2 oz.) per week, since meat is extremely high in saturated fats.

7. Make sure your diet contains adequate **lean protein,** which is essential for proper nutrition, to heal, repair and maintain all of your body's cells and to regulate your basal metabolic rate and to help you lose weight.. As we'll see later, protein is an essential component to the Philly Fit-Step Walking Diet. Some good sources of lean protein are: egg whites; low or non-fat dairy products including cheese, milk, yogurt and soy products; nuts, seeds and beans; fish, poultry without the skin, and lean meats, and whole grain cereals, breads, pastas and noodles.

8. After you've lost all of the weight that you wanted to lose on the Diet-Step® Plan, you are now ready for the **maintenance diet**. You can now increase your intake of total fats slowly every day without gaining an ounce. Concentrate on the **heart-healthy monounsaturated fats,** like nuts and seeds; avocados; fatty fish; olive, peanut and canola oils; low fat dairy products including low fat cheeses, tofu and yogurt. The maintenance diet varies with each individual, depending on height, weight, body build and your own individual metabolism. Some people can maintain their weight on 40 grams of fat daily, while others will be able to maintain their weight by increasing their fat intake to 45 or 50 grams of total fat daily. If you start to gain weight after you've increased your total fat intake, then cut back to 40 grams of total fat daily.

Rebound weight gain does not occur on the Diet-Step®
Maintenance Plan, because by keeping the amount of dietary
fiber the same at 40 grams or more daily, you in effect subdue
the brain's hunger center (appestat). In other words, the more
fiber you eat, the less weight you'll gain. Fiber fills you up
without filling you out.

9. Remember to **eliminate all refined foods** (sugar, flour and
    white rice) and packaged and processed foods and commer-
    cially baked goods). **Also** limit the amount of **salt** which can
    cause fluid retention and can lead to hypertension, and **caf-
    feine** which can stimulate your appetite and cause anxiety,
    palpitations and even high blood pressure). Limit alcohol
    beverages to no more than 3 times per week, since alcohol
    adds additional calories to your diet, (4 ounces red wine or
    12 ounces light beer). Red wine is actually healthier than any
    other alcoholic beverage, since it contains the powerful anti-
    oxidant, resveratrol.

10. Enjoy at least 2-3 servings from the **fruit groups** and 2-3 serv-
    ings from the **vegetable groups** each day which helps to con-
    trol your appetite on the Diet-Step plan. For a wide variety of
    nutrients, choose fruits and vegetables in a rainbow of colors.
    As you'll see in Chapter 3, these fruits and vegetables contain
    many disease fighting phyto-nutrients, vitamins and minerals
    which may reduce the risk of some cancers and help to prevent
    heart disease.

11. Choose from an array of **high-fiber, nutritious, complex
    carbohydrates** that fill you up without filling you out. These
    foods provide high-octane fuel to power you through the day
    and keep you energized for physical activity. The following
    foods are excellent sources of fiber: barley, oats, bran, wheat
    germ, bulgur and brown rice; beans, peas and lentils; whole-
    grain breads and pastas; and most fruits and vegetables includ-
    ing apples, broccoli, brussels sprouts, berries, cabbage, carrots,

grapefruit, oranges, pears, plums, prunes, raisins and spinach, among others (see Fat & Fiber Counter in the Appendix).

12. Also remember to drink at least **six 8 oz. glasses of water daily.** Recent medical studies have shown that drinking a lot of **artificially flavored drinks**, like diet sodas, can actually increase your appetite due to the artificial sweeteners present in these drinks. So be careful not to overuse diet sodas. Switch to unsweetened ice tea or lemonade or just plain water or seltzer.

13. Don't forget to **walk 40 minutes every day except Sunday** or any other day in the week that you'd like to rest. Two 20 minute walks work just as well.

14. When you start to formulate your own meal combinations of 40 grams fat/40 grams fiber, you can keep a daily record of the total grams of fat and the total grams of fiber that you eat at each meal. Make sure that the total for each day adds up to no more than 40 grams of total fat and no less than 40 grams of fiber. You can record these meal plans on 3 x 5 file cards, on your computer, or on your smart phone. Choose any method that's easy, convenient and fun for you. If you're not interested in recording your meals, then just add them up mentally ever day by consulting the Fat & Fiber Counter at the end of the book. You will lose weight quickly and easily on The Philly Fit-Step® Walking Diet, without worrying about rebound weight gain. The weight you lose will stay lost forever.

LOSE UP TO 15 POUNDS & 3 INCHES IN ONLY 21 DAYS

You can lose up to **15 lbs. & 3 inches in only 21 days** on the quick weight-loss formula and easily fit back into your jeans. It is more than likely that your weight-loss will taper off slightly after the first three weeks on the diet as your body's metabolism adjusts to this diet and walking weight-loss program. Remember to keep up with your 40 minute or two 20 minute walking sessions, six days every week. If you'd like to lose weight even more quickly, then consult (Chapter 7: DIETWALK: Quick Weight-Loss).

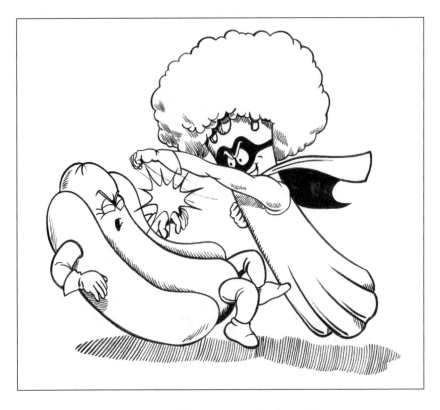

"Philly Fiber to the Rescue."

3

PHILLY FIBER: SECRET AGENT

The Philly Fit-Step Walking Diet has a secret agent working somewhere in Philadelphia, known only as **Philly Fiber**. He is actually a secret agent working behind the scenes for the good people of Philadelphia. This super fiber secret agent blocks fat and burns calories for weight-loss, and also contains a multitude of healthy ingredients that prevent many degenerative diseases, including heart disease, high blood pressure, strokes and even some forms of cancer. This fiber agent actually helps us to live longer, healthier lives. Philly Fiber is truly a hero, since he is a secret agent for weight-loss, good health, and fitness.

Fiber is the general term for those parts of plant food that we are unable to digest. Approximately 15% of the starch in foods (known as resistant starch) is tightly bound to fiber and resists the normal digestive processes. Bacteria normally present in the colon ferment this resistant starch and change it into short-chain fatty acids, which are important to normal bowel health and may also help to protect the colon from cancer-causing agents. Foods that contain resistant starch include breads, cereals, pasta, rice, potatoes and legumes

Fiber is not found in foods of animal origin (meats and dairy products). Plant foods contain a mixture of different types of fibers. These fibers can be divided into soluble or insoluble depending on their solubility in water.

1. **Insoluble fibers:** (cellulose, hemi-celluloses, lignin) make up the structural parts of the cell walls of plants. These fibers absorb many times their own weight in water, creating a soft bulk to the stool and hasten the passage of waste products out of the body. These insoluble fibers promote bowel regularity and aid in the prevention and treatment of some forms of constipation, hemorrhoids, and diverticulitis. These insoluble fibers also may decrease the risk of colon cancer by diluting potentially harmful substances, particularly bile acids, which can cause inflammation and pre-cancerous changes in the lining of the wall of the colon.

2. **Soluble fibers**: (gums, pectins, and mucilages) are found with-in the plant cells. These fibers form a gel, which slows both stomach emptying and absorption of simple sugars from the intestines. This process helps to regulate blood sugar levels, which is particularly helpful in diabetic patients and is helpful in controlling weight in non-diabetics. Many soluble fibers can also assist in lowering blood cholesterol by binding with bile acids and cholesterol and eliminating the cholesterol through the intestinal tract before the cholesterol can be absorbed into the blood stream. These soluble fibers actually form a fiber network, like a spider's web, around fatty foods and carry them out of the intestines before they have a chance to be absorbed. Less fat absorbed, means lower blood cholesterol and less fat deposited in your body's fat cells. The best sources of soluble fiber are fruits and vegetables, oat bran, barley, dried peas and beans, flax and psyllium seeds.

Neither of these types of fiber is digestible in the sense that they provide nutritional value. Insoluble fiber remains more intact as it passes through the intestines, whereas water soluble fiber forms a gel-like substance in the intestines. Each type of fiber is important for health and helpful in preventing weight gain.

HOW FIBER HELPS YOU LOSE WEIGHT

Weight control is aided by the slower emptying of the stomach when you ingest soluble fibers. This causes a feeling of fullness and a decrease in hunger, causing fewer calories to be consumed. For example, if you eat an apple, which has high fiber content, you'll have a feeling of fullness, as compared to eating a cupcake, which has no fiber, and which is the same weight and size as the apple. In fact, it would take approximately three cupcakes to satisfy your brain's hunger center before you realized that you were full. Well, by then you would already have consumed 480 calories, 12 grams of sugar, and 17 grams of fat.

A. Fiber helps in weight loss and weight control by the simple fact that high-fiber foods contain **fewer calories for their large volume.** Fiber-rich foods, such as fruits and vegetables, whole-grain cereals and breads, potatoes and legumes are low in fat calories and have a high water content. You are eating less and enjoying it more.

B. High fiber foods have a **high bulk ratio**, which satisfies the hunger center more quickly than low fiber foods; consequently, fewer calories are consumed. Fiber-rich foods take longer to chew and to digest than fiber-depleted foods, which, in turn gives your stomach time to feel full. When you feel full earlier you eat less.

C. The following carbohydrate foods have a **low glycemic index**, and for all intents and purposes can be labeled as good high fiber carbs:

 • Most vegetables, with the exception of corn and white potatoes.

 • Most fruits with the skin intact, with the exception of fruit juices, which contain high levels of sugar and very little actual fruit. Some fruits, for example, watermelon and grapes, do have a high sugar content and have to be consumed in moderation.

- Beans and legumes are excellent sources of fiber, protein, vitamins, minerals, and nutrients.

- Whole grains.

- Whole-grain cereals, such as oatmeal (instant oatmeal may have a high sugar content) or cold cereals are good choices for low glycemic carbohydrates. Make sure that the package shows a fiber count of, at least, 5 to 6 grams of fiber per serving, and a sugar count lower than 10 to 12 grams of sugar per serving, preferably less than 8 grams.

- Whole-grain breads. The first ingredient listed on the label of whole-grain breads should be "whole grain flour." If it doesn't list whole-grain flour first, then it is really not whole-grain bread. This includes any type of whole-grain bread products.

- Brown long-grain rice makes a good low glycemic addition to any meal, since it is broken down and absorbed slowly.

- Whole wheat pastas now come in many varieties, such as noodles, spaghetti, vermicelli, linguini, etc.

- Nuts are good low glycemic snack foods. In addition to being absorbed slowly, they are excellent sources of protein, fiber, magnesium, copper, folic acid, potassium, and vitamin D. Nuts are also considered "the good fats," which are actually called monounsaturated fats. They help to keep the blood vessels open, which, in turn, can reduce the risk of heart disease and strokes. Raw nuts, in particular, are called "heart healthy" nuts, since they contain generous amounts of omega-3 fatty acids. These omega-3 fatty acids are heart protective, and have also been known to prevent certain forms of cancer.

D. A high-fiber diet is essentially a **healthy, low-fat diet**, which decreases the intake of refined and processed food. This encourages the consumption of fresh fruits, vegetables, and whole-grain cereals and breads. When the fiber is eaten from any of the food sources, it produces its most beneficial effect when it is eaten with each meal of the day. Dietary fiber takes longer to chew and eat, with the subsequent development of more saliva and a larger bulk swallowing effect with each mouthful. The larger bulk helps to fill the stomach and causes a decrease in hunger before more calories can be consumed. High-fiber diets help to provide bulk without energy and may reduce the amount of energy absorbed from the food that is eaten. These high-fiber diets are often referred to as having a low-energy density and appear to prevent excessive caloric (energy) intake. Countries that consume high-fiber diets rarely have obesity problems. Philly's Fit-Step Walking Diet incorporates at least 40 grams or more of fiber into its diet for good health and weight-loss.

Good Carbs

High fiber, good carbs **burn more calories** during digestion and make you feel fuller earlier and longer than eating refined bad carbs. These good carbs have **a low glycemic index** and are absorbed slowly and cause only a moderate rise in blood sugar and insulin levels. This even level of insulin can *slowly process the blood sugar into the body's cells for energy production,* and there is no rapid filling of the cells with fat caused by high levels of sugar and insulin surges, which in turn causes binge carbohydrate eating. Most vegetables (except corn and white potatoes), fruits (not fruit juices), beans, nuts, legumes, chick peas, whole-grain cereals and breads fall into this category. The good carbs are primarily of plant origin and are naturally low in fat and calories, and contain phyto-nutrients, vitamins, minerals, enzymes and fiber.

These good carbs are helpful in a weight-loss program, because your body slowly converts these good carbs into glucose in the intestinal tract, which is then slowly absorbed into the blood stream. This slow absorption of glucose then causes the pancreas to produce insulin at a steady even level, which results in normal levels of blood sugar and insulin in your blood stream. Therefore, there is no rapid filling of the fat cells with excess sugar, because there are no spikes in insulin and sugar levels. This results in your appetite being nicely controlled and prevents you from gaining excess weight.

When you consume good carbs (complex carbohydrates) that have a low glycemic index, your body expends 2½ times more energy converting these good carbs from your intestinal tract into your blood stream into energy stores than it does converting bad carbs or fat into energy. This means that a high-fiber, complex carbohydrate, low-fat diet causes your body to work that much harder after each meal, burning more calories to produce energy. This in turn boosts your basal metabolic rate which results in the additional burning of about 250 extra calories by the simple thermic action of converting carbohydrates into energy. This means that you are not only consuming fewer calories by eating good carbs but you are actually burning additional calories just by the simple process of eating and digesting these good carbs. A really neat trick!

Good carbs include whole grain cereals and breads, fresh fruits and vegetables, beans and lentils, sweet potatoes and brown rice, hummus (chick peas) and popcorn (whole grain corn kernels). Many of the whole grain cereals and whole grain bread products contain fiber as well as some protein. When you refine whole grain foods, you remove both the fiber and the protein content by up to 50%.

Both fiber and protein help to curb your appetite by helping you feel fuller earlier in the course of your meal. This fiber-protein combo slows the rate at which your body absorbs this combination of protein and fiber, thus, minimizing blood sugar and insulin spikes, which can otherwise stimulate your appetite. Also by preventing the production of excess insulin, this fiber-protein combo prevents fat from being deposited in your fat cells, particularly those fat cells located in your abdominal wall. So in effect, you are melting away belly fat as you consume this important fiber-protein combination.

By increasing the lean protein content and decreasing the fat content of your meals, you can slowly and safely lose weight that will stay permanently lost. Unlike low-carb diets, you won't experience rapid rebound weight gain that invariably occurs when you stop the diet, and you'll avoid the nasty side effects and hidden health problems inherent in these unsafe low-carb diets. All low carb diets are high-fat diets and the excess fat calories you eat are stored in your fat cells indefinitely. Complex carbs on the other hand cause your body to work harder during digestion, burning more calories for immediate energy production and for **glycogen** storage in your muscles and liver (which is actually *stored energy*) for use at a later time.

BAD CARBS & GLYCEMIC INDEX

Foods with **low-fiber content** are, in most cases, considerably **more concentrated in calories.** The main element which differentiates bad carbs from good carbs is how fast the carbohydrate foods are converted into sugar in the intestine and absorbed into the bloodstream. This rapid increase in blood sugar causes a rapid increase in **insulin levels** which in turn causes you to become hungry sooner because of the drop in blood sugar. Excessive calories are then consumed and excess insulin is produced causing the *body fat cells to store more fat*, because the production of **glycogen** (stored energy in muscles and liver) is inhibited, which normally causes the body's fat cells to burn stored fuel). Fat cells therefore store more fat instead of burning fat for the production of energy, Result: **Less energy produced, more fat stored**.

The Glycemic Index was developed in order to measure carbohydrate foods' effects on blood sugar levels. White flour and white rice, refined highly-processed flour (white breads, cereals, spaghetti, bagels, muffins, pretzels, pancakes), fruit juices and sodas, cakes, pies, ice cream, cookies, candies, chips, and soda have a high-glycemic index, which means that once they pass through the intestinal tract, they are quickly absorbed and cause a rapid spike in blood glucose and insulin levels. Then the rapidly fluctuating glucose and insulin levels lead to excessive calories being consumed, which have no place to go except to be stored in your body's fat cells. This invariably leads to excessive weight gain. High-glycemic diets increase the risk of diabetes, heart disease, strokes and certain forms of cancer. High fiber foods such as whole grain cereals and breads have a low-glycemic index, which causes only a gradual rise in blood sugar and insulin levels. These low-glycemic index foods reduce the risk of developing heart disease and diabetes.

The increased insulin levels that are needed to fill the muscle and fat cells with sugar also inhibit the production of a muscle protein called *glucagon,* which is a protein that normally signals the body's fat cells to burn stored fuel when the blood glucose levels fall below a critical level. Since this production of glucagon is inhibited, the fat cells store more fat instead of burning fat for the production of energy. Result: Less energy produced, more fat stored. This is actually the opposite condition that you want to happen.

In addition to gaining unwanted pounds, eating foods with a high glycemic index can cause or contribute to health problems. When excess insulin is repeatedly produced by the pancreas by ingesting high-glycemic foods, the pancreas's insulin-producing cells can actually wear out, and then they begin to produce less and less insulin. This can eventually lead to diabetes. Also, overweight people may develop a condition known as insulin resistance. This is where the body's tissues resist insulin's signal to transfer glucose from the blood into the cells. This is another way that people on high glycemic diets can develop a condition known as *insulin-resistant diabetes.* Exercise and weight reduction are certainly ways that this condition can be prevented.

The bad carbs are:

1. Refined or processed flour (white bread, bagels, muffins, croissants, cakes, pies, pastries, cereals, and refined pastas).

2. Processed snack foods, which include crackers, chips, pretzels, any type of cookies, or potato or corn chips.

3. Sugar-laden desserts, such as cakes, frostings, pies, muffins, ice cream, sorbets, sherbet, sugary drinks like ice tea and lemonade, sports drinks, fruit juices, sodas, and soft drinks, unless labeled as diet or sugar-free.

4. Corn and white potatoes are the only bad carb vegetables.

5. Fruits; only those fruits with high sugar content, such as watermelon and grapes, have a high glycemic index.

These fiber-deficient foods require hardly any chewing and have little or no bulk content. Therefore, large amounts of calories are consumed when eating these foods before your appetite center in the brain (appestat) is satisfied. These low-fiber foods are more concentrated in calories, so that more food must be eaten before the stomach can be filled.

Don't be fooled by the terms: **net-carbs, or non-impact carbs**. These terms are part of a marketing scam to mislead the public. Soluble fiber and sugar alcohol are included in the deducted carbohydrates, when in fact they are part of the total amount of carbohydrates. They need to be included to determine the body's ability to burn fats or store carbs as fats. There have been no studies that prove that low "net-carb" foods help people lose weight, and the FDA does not regulate the term and methods for calculating it.

FIBER BLOCKS FATS AND BURNS CALORIES

Dietary fiber is one of your best foods to block both the absorption of fat and to burn up extra calories. Sounds almost too good to be true; however, it really works. First of all, when you combine the high-fiber foods that we have already discussed, combined with any fat in your diet, like a piece of cake or a hamburger, each gram of fiber traps fat globules by entwining them in a fiber-like web, made up of thousands of fiber strands. Once these fat globules are trapped in the fiber's web, they pass through the intestinal tract before they are absorbed into the bloodstream. Therefore, these fat globules are excreted in the waste material from your colon without getting absorbed and stored as fat in your body. The fiber is actually removing the fat from your body like a garbage truck removes garbage. And to underscore that fact, fat really is garbage.

Secondly, fiber actually burns up calories by itself. This is accomplished because fiber causes your intestinal tract to work harder in order to digest the fiber foods. The body's metabolism uses more energy for this time-consuming digestion, and therefore can actually consume most of the calories that the fiber foods contain. Strange as it seems, some heavily fibered foods can actually burn more calories than the fiber foods actually contain, thereby creating a deficit of calories. This causes the body to use stored body fat for the production of energy. Each gram of fiber that you consume can burn up approximately 9 calories, most of which come from fat. So if you eat 30 grams of fiber a day, you can burn an additional 270 calories daily (30 grams fiber x 9 calories). You can subtract those 270 calories every day from your total daily calorie intake, without actually cutting those calories from your diet.

In addition to blocking fat and burning calories, fiber foods bind with water in the intestinal tract and form bulk that makes you feel full early in the course of your meal. So you eat less, and therefore you consume fewer calories at each meal. Also, your appestat (hunger mechanism) is satisfied for longer periods of time, since it takes longer to digest fiber foods, and therefore you will have less of a tendency to snack between meals.

A RAINBOW OF HEALTHY POWER FOODS

Many recent medical studies have proved that colorful fruits and vegetables and grains, nuts and seeds, contain cancer-fighting substances and can provide a full spectrum of disease prevention. For maximum health benefits, you should eat a variety of vegetables and fruits of many different colors. These colors are formed by pigments in each individual plant. The reason for the different colors is that each colored fruit or vegetable has a different phyto-chemical (phyto means plant). These phyto-chemicals in the fruits and vegetables contain many essential nutrients that help to decrease the risk of heart disease, hypertension, blood clots, degenerative diseases of aging, and certain forms of cancer. It is important to eat at least 4-5 servings of fruit or vegetables per day.

The multiple colors of the spectrum found in various fruits and vegetables are derived from their own individual plant pigment. Each one of these colorful fruits and vegetables offer a full spectrum of disease prevention from the phytonutrients and antioxidants found in each plant's beautiful colors. The Philly Fit-Step Diet Plan contains an abundance of all of these healthy nutrients.

The following is a list of some of the phyto-chemicals and antioxidants present in fruits, vegetables, grains and seeds and nuts that can reduce your risk of many diseases:

Spinach If you're looking for a vegetable with super healing powers, try spinach. It's packed with vitamins, antioxidants, and minerals that will protect you from many diseases. Spinach contains many antioxidants including beta and alpha carotenes, lutein, zeaxanthin, potassium, magnesium, vitamin K and folic acid. Recent studies at two major universities have found that, as strange as it seems, spinach may lower the risk of strokes, colon cancer, cataracts, heart disease, osteoporosis, hip fractures, memory loss, Alzheimer's disease, depression and even birth defects. The disease fighting properties in spinach are better absorbed when spinach is cooked with a little olive oil. Now, that's what I call a power healthy vegetable.

Other dark green leafy vegetables (collard greens, kale, bok choy, mustard greens) are low in calories and have high fiber content. These crunchy foods take longer to chew, which helps to shut off the brain's hunger control mechanism (appestat). Kale and spinach are two vegetables rich in the antioxidants *lutein* and *zeaxanthin*. These antioxidants have been reported to protect against age-related cataracts and macular degeneration, one of the leading causes of blindness. Also high in these vision-protecting antioxidants are romaine lettuce, broccoli, collards, turnip greens, and corn.

Green leafy vegetables are low in calories and are filling because of their fiber content and their crunch factor. Crunchy fiber foods take longer to eat and help your brain's hunger mechanism to shut down quickly. Fiber also helps to prevent the absorption of fat from the intestinal tract by wrapping threads of fiber around the fat globules, thus preventing the fat's absorption into the blood and actually sweeping the fat through and out of the intestinal tract before it is absorbed. Green leafy vegetables also contain many plant nutrients, antioxidants, and B-complex vitamins, which help to prevent cancer, heart disease, and degenerative neurological diseases.

Broccoli and broccoli sprouts contain power nutrients that can reduce your risk of heart disease, and certain types of cancer. The active antioxidant in broccoli is *glucoraphanin*, which has been shown to boost your body's defense mechanism against cancer-causing free radicals that damage normal cells in the body. This particular antioxidant also lowers blood pressure, strengthens the immune system, decreases inflammation in the body and has been shown to reduce the incidence of strokes.

Sweet Potatoes are excellent sources of folic acid, beta-carotene, potassium, vitamins A, C, B-complex, and beta-carotene. These nutrients combined with sweet potatoes plant sterols can decrease your risk of heart disease. They are a great addition to any weight-loss program because of their high fiber content and their nutritional value. These nutrients combined with plant sterols, found in sweet potatoes, are powerful antioxidants, which can help to lower cholesterol and lower your risk of heart disease. When sweet potatoes are eaten with their skin, they are good sources of both insoluble and soluble fiber. These two types of fibers help to reduce your appetite the way most fiber foods do, by filling you up and satisfying your appetite early, without supplying extra calories in your diet.

Tomatoes contain the antioxidant lycopene which helps to prevent both prostate and breast cancers. Tomatoes also contain lots of vitamin C, which when combined with *lycopene* can help to lower your blood cholesterol.

Tomatoes are unique in their ability to produce an amino acid called *carnitine.* This amino acid causes your body to burn fat at a faster rate by increasing your body's basal metabolic rate. Any tomato products, from ketchup to tomato sauce, are great for your weight-reducing diet.

Asparagus is an excellent source of potassium, folic acid, beta-carotene, vitamin C, and the antioxidant *glutathione*, which helps to fight nasty free radicals, which can damage normal cells. Asparagus is a great addition to any diet program, since it is low in calories and high in nutrients. Steamed asparagus is great eaten alone or in a salad. It must be refrigerated or frozen quickly to prevent the loss of its nutritional value. If boiled too long, most of the nutrients end up in the water.

Beans are high in potassium and low in sodium, which helps to reduce your risk of developing high blood pressure and strokes. Beans are chock full of fiber, which helps to reduce the absorption of fat and unwanted calories from the gastro-intestinal tract. The high fiber content of beans is great for your weight loss plan, since it reduces your appetite by filling you up faster, so that you eat fewer calories. Beans have almost as many calories and as much protein as meat without the added saturated fat. The fiber and water content of beans make you feel fuller earlier in your meal so that you don't consume excess calories. One cup of cooked beans (⅔ of a can) contains 12 grams of fiber whereas meat contains no fiber at all. Meat is therefore digested quickly whereas fiber is digested slowly, keeping you satisfied longer. Beans are also low in sugar, which prevents insulin from spiking in the bloodstream and causing hunger pangs.

In a recent study, bean eaters weighed on average, seven pounds less and had slimmer waists than their bean-avoiding counterparts, even though they consumed 200 calories less daily than the non-bean eaters. Beans also contain antioxidants and phytonutrients which fight dangerous free-radicals in your body, which can cause degenerative diseases of aging, cardiovascular diseases, and cancer. The beans that contain the most antioxidants are: red kidney beans, pinto beans, small red beans, navy beans, black beans, and black-eyed peas. Beans have lots of fiber and protein and no fat at all. This is the perfect combination for a super power food.

Peas are packed with vitamins A, B-1, B-6, C, and vitamin K, which are known for maintaining strong bones and helping blood to clot in order to prevent bleeding. Peas are high in fiber and are an excellent source of vegetable protein. They also have the added benefit of containing no fat or cholesterol. One cup of peas, which contains approximately 100 calories, has as much protein as a tablespoon of peanut butter or a ¼ cup of nuts. Peas are another example of a super power food even though they're very small. Size doesn't really matter. Other vegetables that are rich sources of Vitamin K are: cabbage, broccoli, spinach, cauliflower, and beans.

Peppers are great sources of vitamins A, C, B-complex, beta-carotene, folic acid, and potassium. All colors of sweet peppers (red, yellow, green) are high in fiber and low in calories and are great foods for your Fit-Step Diet weight-loss plan. Peppers contain spices that also can reduce your appetite because they satisfy your taste buds and hunger before you've had a chance to eat a big meal. Peppers also have antioxidants that help to prevent strokes and heart attacks by decreasing the blood platelets stickiness, thus preventing blood clots from forming.

Hot peppers contain higher quantities of antioxidants than sweet peppers. They also contain phytonutrients that help to prevent certain forms of cancer. Hot peppers also contain an ingredient called *capsaicin*, which makes these peppers hot and spicy. This ingredient has anti-inflammatory properties and helps to relieve the pain of various forms of arthritis and nerve inflammations. These capsaicinoids can cause eye irritation if transferred from your hands to your eyes, so be careful to wash your hands thoroughly after handling hot peppers.

Soybeans contain soy proteins, which help reduce the risk of cardiovascular disease. The reason for this is that soy proteins reduce the amount of total fat and LDL cholesterol in the blood by affecting the synthesis and metabolism of cholesterol in the liver. Its amino acid composition differs from the structure of other proteins found in meat and milk. Clinical trials showed a significantly lower incidence of coronary heart disease in patients with a high soy intake. Soybeans can be found in many different varieties, including soy beverages, tofu, tempeh, soy-based meat substitutes, and some baked goods. However, to qualify, such soy-rich foods should contain at least 6.5 grams of soy protein, and less than 3 grams of total fat per serving and less than 1 gram of saturated fat per serving in order to qualify as a heart healthy food. One-half cup of cooked soybeans contains 4 grams of fiber. Soybeans are also a good source of dietary fiber.

In another related study, soy supplements were shown to cut the risk of developing colon cancer in half. Soy supplements also decreased the relative risk of having a recurrence of colon cancer in high-risk subjects. This study was reported at the annual conference of The American Institute for Cancer Research. High soy intake may be able to delay the onset of colon cancer in those at risk, or may lead to more cancer-free years in those whose initial cancer was surgically removed.

Soy contains natural phytonutrients called *isoflavones*. These plant chemicals break down the fat which is stored in your body's fat cells. Several studies have confirmed that the consumption of soy products on a regular basis helps dieters' burn fat and lose weight without any other alteration in their diets. These isoflavones present in soy also have been shown to reduce the incidence of heart disease. In addition to helping you lose weight by breaking down the stored fat in your body, isoflavones also break down saturated fat in your blood, thus lowering the LDL bad cholesterol. Soy products (soy milk, soy yogurt, tofu, etc.) are good for your heart and great for your figure.

Mushrooms: Many types of mushrooms contain the amino acid *glutamic acid*, which boosts the immune system and helps to fight various types of infections. By helping to improve the body's immune system, mushrooms have also been known to fight certain forms of cancer and autoimmune diseases, such as rheumatoid arthritis, lupus, and other collagen disease. Mushrooms are also rich in potassium and vitamin C, which help to keep blood pressure normal.

Portobello and white mushrooms have a high content of certain nutrients and minerals, particularly *selenium*, which may help to reduce the risk of prostate and breast cancer. When selenium is combined with the vitamin E present in mushrooms, it helps to prevent nasty free radicals from damaging the body's normal cells, thus slowing the aging process. Shiitake mushrooms also contain many plant nutrients, in particular *lentinan* and *eritadenine*, which help to improve the immune system and assist in lowering blood cholesterol. These phytonutrients have also been shown to reduce the risk of heart disease and certain forms of cancer.

All mushrooms are low in calories and are fat-free, making them excellent staples in a weight-loss program. They are excellent flavor enhancers for a variety of foods. Mushrooms are not only good for you, but they are great for your weight-loss program.

Onions and Curry: In a recent study from Johns Hopkins University School of Medicine, it was found that the chemicals found in onions and curry may help to prevent colon cancer. The antioxidant found in onions is called *quercetin*, and the antioxidant found in curry is called *curcumin*. It is thought that these two powerful antioxidants decrease the formation of colon polyps in patients who have an inherited-type of precancerous colon polyps. The average number of polyps decreased by 60% and the average size of the polyps decreased by 50% in patients who consumed these two powerful antioxidants found in both onions and curry.

Grapefruit contains high levels of potassium, vitamin C, beta-carotene, and the antioxidant *lycopene*, which has been shown to reduce the risk of both breast and prostate cancers. Grapefruits also contain bioflavonoids, which appear to protect against heart disease. They also contain phytonutrients, which include *phenolic acid*, which can block nitrosamines, which are cancer-causing chemicals found in many smoked foods.

Grapefruits are a great addition to any weight-reduction program, since they are low in calories and high in fiber. The only precaution is that patients who are on cholesterol-lowering drugs called the statins should be careful about drinking grapefruit juice with these medications. Grapefruit juice appears to slow the natural breakdown of these drugs in the bloodstream, causing higher than expected levels of these medications to stay active in the blood for longer periods of time. Check with your doctor about eating grapefruit if you are taking statins.

Oranges protect your heart and fight cancer. A recent study showed that oranges boost HDL cholesterol, in addition to providing vitamin C, folic acid, and numerous flavonoids. These compounds are thought to prevent cholesterol oxidation, which has been linked to a reduced risk of coronary events. An orange or two a day will keep atherosclerosis away. Researchers have found that citrus fruits, in particular oranges, also showed anti-cancer activity in animals and in test tubes. These researchers found that animals that ate oranges for several months were 25% less likely to develop early colon cancer than animals given only water. Compounds such as *liminoids* in oranges seem to alter the characteristics of the colon lining, discouraging cancer growth. These researchers speculate that oranges not orange juice may also help to suppress breast cancer, prostate, and lung cancer

Apples: The old adage that, "an apple a day keeps the doctor away," may contain more truth than we actually realize. When you eat an apple with the skin on it every day, you help prevent many health related problems. Apples contain an antioxidant called *Quercetin* which has many beneficial properties. First of all this compound acts as an antihistamine which may help to relieve the symptoms of asthma and other allergy related problems. Quercetin also has anti-inflammatory properties that may reduce the pain associated with arthritis and other inflammatory problems. This unique antioxidant has also been shown to protect the brain cells from circulatory damage, which can help to prevent strokes and reduce the incidence of age-related neurological disorders such as Alzheimer's disease. And finally, this nutrient found in apples has been shown to lower blood cholesterol and helps to keep your lungs healthy. It has also been shown to reduce the incidence of certain forms of cancer, including breast and prostate cancer.

Apples, because of their high water and pectin fiber content will help you to lose weight by providing bulk to your diet, which controls your brain's appetite control mechanism. Apples also help to fight inflammation in the muscles of the body which can cause an increase in the enzyme *CRP (C-reactive protein)*. This enzyme may be responsible for heart attacks, and some forms of arthritis.

The two types of fiber present in apples help to prevent the formation of cholesterol deposits in your arteries and the development of blood clots in your bloodstream. Several studies have proven that eating apples lowered the bad cholesterol (LDL) in your bloodstream which contributed to fatal heart attacks and strokes. This high fiber content also helps to prevent the quick absorption of glucose into the bloodstream, which in turn limits high spikes in insulin levels. This factor has been attributed to a lower risk of developing obesity and diabetes.

Apples also increase the body's production of *Acetylcholine*, which has a beneficial effect on mental acuity and memory. They also contain another antioxidant called *Apigenin*, which appears to decrease the number of attacks in asthmatic patients.

Blueberries may reverse aging process. New research has indicated that women on antioxidant-rich diets showed fewer age-related disorders than those on a normal diet. The studies showed that among all the fruits and vegetables, the benefits were greatest with blueberries, which reversed age-related effects; for example, loss of balance and lack of coordination. They also discovered that blueberry extract had the greatest effect on reversing aging decline. Antioxidants help neutralize free radical by-products on the conversion of oxygen into energy, which, if not neutralized, can cause oxidative stress and lead to cell damage. Previous studies have shown that both strawberries and spinach extract can also help to prevent the onset of age-related defects. However, the greatest effect was shown in patients who ate blueberries. Phytonutrients in blueberries, particularly flavonoids and beta-carotene, seem to have an anti-inflammatory effect, which may even help in the prevention of Alzheimer's disease. Again, we have another solid recommendation for eating fruits and vegetables because of their high fiber content and because of their phytonutrients and antioxidants.

Fruits and vegetables in general contain various healthy antioxidants and phytonutrients that prevent many cardiovascular and degenerative diseases of aging, including several forms of cancer. New studies have also shown that fruits can prevent or reduce the incidence of uterine fibroids, which are the most commonly diagnosed uterine tumors. These tumors have been associated with anemia, pelvic pain, and in some cases, fertility problems. It appears that women who have high levels of estrogens, which may be related to high meat intake, are more prone to fibroids. A recent study showed that diets decreasing or eliminating meats and increasing green vegetables have a significant effect on the prevention of the development of fibroids. The vegetables and fruits contain *isoflavinoids*, which can offset the effect of estrogen on the body. Also, by eliminating meat from the diet, the levels of estrogen in the body decrease. By decreasing meat and increasing fiber, the body is less likely to develop estrogen-related uterine fibroid tumors.

Veggies and fruits also help prevent breast and uterine cancer. Women who limit their intake of red meat and eat lots of green vegetables have a reduced risk of developing breast cancer and uterine cancer. High levels of estrogen, which results from the consumption of beef, ham, pork, and other red meat, have been implicated in the formation of breast and uterine cancer. The intake of 4-5 servings of fruits and vegetables daily with phytonutrients, in particular, isoflavinoids, may offset some of estrogen's effect on the uterus and breast.

Cruciferous vegetables also decrease risk of bladder cancer. In a recent study on bladder cancer, it was shown that in order to reduce the risk of bladder cancer, it is necessary to drink lots of fluids, not to smoke, and to eat lots of cruciferous vegetables. A high intake of cruciferous vegetables, particularly broccoli and cabbage, significantly reduced the risk of bladder cancer. This may be explained by the presence of one or more phytochemicals in broccoli and cabbage, which are specific in the reduction of bladder cancer risk. This study also showed that a high intake of fruits, yellow vegetables, and green, leafy vegetables did not significantly reduce the risk of bladder cancer. The relationship with high cruciferous vegetable intake (broccoli and cabbage) was associated with the highest reduction in the risk of developing bladder cancer.

Nuts have a low glycemic index and are absorbed slowly. They are also a good source of protein and contain many essential nutrients such as fiber, copper, magnesium, folic acid, vitamin D, E, and potassium. Nuts, particularly walnuts and almonds, contain heart-healthy monounsaturated fats. These good fats can lower blood cholesterol, prevent heart disease and reduce the incidence of high blood pressure.

Nuts actually help to retain the natural elasticity of the blood vessels, which helps to lower blood pressure. Nuts, especially walnuts, have a high content of an amino acid called *L-argentine* and also contain *alpha-linoline acid*, which is a plant-based omega-3 fatty acid. These two compounds help to dilate your arteries and offer additional heart-protective properties as well as to help prevent certain forms of cancer.

Nuts are also an excellent source of protein, which acts as a natural appetite suppressant, because of its slow digestion and absorption into the blood stream. Most of the energy contained in the protein in nuts is burned as fuel for all of your body's metabolic function. Therefore, hardly any of the calories contained in the dietary protein found in nuts is converted into fat storage, which is why nuts are a good addition to the Fit-Step Diet weight-loss plan.

Frequent consumption of walnuts (four to five servings per week) has been shown to reduce the risk of coronary heart disease by as much as 50%. Nuts also have been shown to decrease both the total cholesterol by 5-10% and the LDL cholesterol by 15-20%. A study published in *The Journal of Nutrition* indicated that of all edible plants, walnuts have one of the highest concentrations of antioxidants. In a more recent study reported in the *Journal of Circulation,* from the Hospital Clinic of Barcelona, Spain, Dr. Emilio Ros said that, "This is the first time a whole food, not its isolated components, has shown this beneficial effect on vascular health." He further stated that, "Walnuts differ from all other nuts because of their high content of alpha-linolenic acid (ALA), a plant-based omega-3 fatty acid, which may provide additional heart-protective properties." Several other beneficial components of walnuts include: L-arginine, which may be cardio protective by dilating the arteries. Walnuts also contain fiber, folic acid, gamma-tocopherol, and other antioxidants, which also help to prevent atherosclerosis (hardening of the arteries).

Whole grains: In a recent study in the *American Journal of Clinical Nutrition*, women who ate three to four servings of whole grains a day had one-third to one-half the risk of developing heart disease as opposed to women who ate refined flour, such as white bread.

It is important to check the ingredients in any commercial food to see that it is truly made from whole grains. In particular, it is important to check the ingredients in snack foods (for example, cookies, crackers, and chips), since many of these products contain not only refined white flour, but also partially hydrogenated oils (trans-fats), which actually can raise our cholesterol more than other types of saturated fats.

Recent studies have subsequently shown that high fiber diets, which include not only cereal grains, but fruits and vegetables, do, indeed, help to prevent against the development of colon cancer. As part of the ongoing Nurses' Health Study, their report showed that women who ate a diet high in red meat had higher rates of colorectal cancer. In that same study, women whose diets were low in red meat and high in fruits, vegetables, and cereal grains had a significantly decreased risk of colon cancer. In countries where diets are high in plant-based foods and low in red meat and animal fat, people have lower rates of heart disease and colon cancer.

Oatmeal has a high content of insoluble fiber, which makes it an excellent food for your Fit-Step Diet plan. Insoluble fiber helps to shut off your appetite control mechanism, so oatmeal is absorbed slowly from the intestinal tract. Oatmeal also has a high soluble fiber content, which helps to increase the good (HDL) cholesterol which in turn flushes out the bad (LDL) cholesterol from your blood stream. Oatmeal and other high fiber, bran cereals are also loaded with the mineral magnesium, which helps to regulate your insulin levels and reduces your risk of developing diabetes and obesity.

Oatmeal for breakfast every day has been recommended by the American Heart Association as a great start for your day to reduce your risk of heart disease. People who eat oatmeal, as well as other whole-grain bran-type cereals daily, have less than one-half the risk of developing obesity and diabetes as non-cereal eaters. High-fiber bran cereals help to regulate insulin production in the morning. This helps to control your appetite and reduce the risk of gaining unwanted pounds. Bran cereals are also packed with magnesium, which is a mineral that can also reduce your risk of developing diabetes. Magnesium also helps to stabilize your blood sugar by preventing the overproduction of insulin by the pancreas. Fiber-rich oatmeal is nutritious, tastes great, and is slow to digest. Oatmeal has also been shown to reduce your craving for high-refined sugar products and fatty foods.

THE TOP HIGH-FIBER, ANTIOXIDANT POWER FOODS

FRUITS	VEGGIES	OTHER
Apples	Broccoli	Garlic
Apricots	Bok Choy	Ginger
Blueberries	Cabbage	Nuts
Blackberries	Carrots	Olive oil
Cantaloupe	Cauliflower	Soy beans
Cherries	Greens (others)	Tea
Cranberries	Kale	Whole grains
Mangoes	Spinach	
Mangos	Spinach	
Oranges	Squash	
Prunes	Sweet potatoes	
Purple grapes	Tomatoes	
Raisins		
Raspberries		
Strawberries		

THE MEDITERRANEAN DIET

Research shows that the Mediterranean diet, which emphasizes whole grains, greens, fruits, vegetables, fish and olive oil, is healthier than the typical American diet, which is high in fat and processed foods. There is a significantly decreased risk of heart disease and cancer in the Mediterranean cultures, which have been thriving on these foods for thousands of years. The Mediterranean diet has been found to help protect against heart disease and help to control blood cholesterol and blood sugar levels. In the Mediterranean diet, people consume at least 25-30 grams of fiber a day. In addition to fiber, this diet is rich in **omega-3 fatty acids** from fish oils and **alpha-linoleic acid** from plant sources. Both of these substances help to reduce the incidence of heart disease, The Mediterranean diet is far superior to our western diet, and shows us why fiber is a significantly important factor in their diet.

The Mediterranean diet is rich in **olive oil**, which is a heart-healthy monounsaturated fat that helps to increase your body's good cholesterol (HDL) and decrease the bad cholesterol (LDL). This decreases your risk of heart attacks and strokes by decreasing cholesterol deposits in your arteries. The Mediterranean people use olive oil on almost everything they eat (pastas, breads, salads, vegetables, fish) and even pastries are made with olive oil. They also use olives abundantly in their salads and with their main courses. These people also eat considerably less saturated fat than most countries, including the United States.

And the Mediterranean people have one more secret besides their diet that keeps them healthy and free of many of the diseases of aging. If you haven't guessed it by now, you will certainly discover it later in this book. It's **walking**, of course. Mediterranean people, in addition to eating healthy, walk all of the time. They walk to work, to visit friends, to shop or just to take a carefree walk. Walking is just a natural part of their lives. They seldom drive anywhere unless absolutely necessary. This essential factor is the basic exercise component of *The Philly Fit-Step® Walking Diet.*

In a recent edition of the *Journal American Medical Association*, it was reported that elderly people who followed the Mediterranean diet (olive oil, nuts, seeds, whole grains, vegetables, greens, fish and fruit) and walked 30-40 minutes every day, had a 65% lower mortality rate than a similar age group of people who ate a typical American high fat, low fiber diet and were also sedentary. These individuals who followed the Mediterranean diet had a significant decrease in body weight, blood cholesterol and triglycerides, blood pressure, blood sugar, and insulin levels. They also had a significant increase in their good cholesterol (HDL) and a decrease in their bad cholesterol (LDL), both of which help to decrease the risk of heart disease and strokes. This particular study followed over 2,500 men and women, ages 70-90, in 11 different European countries for a period of 12 years.

In a similar study also reported in the *Journal American Medical Association*, it was found that people on the Mediterranean diet, reduced their risk of developing the **metabolic syndrome.** This condition occurs when excess amounts of fat accumulate around the abdomen because of the body's resistance to insulin due to a high fat, low fiber diet. This syndrome increases a person's risk for developing hypertension, coronary heart disease, diabetes, obesity, certain forms of cancer, and dementia. It was found that the Mediterranean diet actually changed the body chemistry by reducing insulin abnormalities and also by decreasing chronic inflammation in the arteries and other tissues in the body.

FIBER AND CRP

CRP or C-reactive protein is a measure of inflammation that occurs in your body if you have heart disease, high blood pressure, diabetes, or obesity. Adults with these medical conditions, who had a low fiber intake, are two to three times as likely to have an elevated CRP level compared with people who had none of these conditions. There is considerable medical evidence that dietary fiber reduces both inflammation in the body and also reduces blood cholesterol levels.

According to a study conducted by the North American Primary Care Research Group, individuals who had two or more conditions (diabetes, high blood pressure, or obesity) and consumed 20 or more grams of dietary fiber daily, had significantly lower levels of CRP as opposed to those people who consumed eight or less grams of dietary fiber per day. CRP levels were actually four times higher in people with these medical conditions who consumed less than eight grams of fiber daily.

The American Heart Association and the American Diabetes Association both recommend that adults should consume at least 30 to 35 grams of fiber per day. So in addition to its long line of health benefits (lower blood pressure, low heart disease risk, low cholesterol levels, improved GI function, weight control, etc.), fiber now has the unique distinction of lowering the levels of a very dangerous component in the blood, namely c-reactive protein. CRP also may actually be implicated in contributing to other degenerative diseases of aging including arthritis and cancer.

FIBER: REDUCES STROKES & HEART ATTACKS

At the annual scientific session of the American Heart Association, it was found that people who ate more fruit and vegetables had reduced rates of cardiovascular diseases. It was found that every portion of fruits and vegetables eaten per day improves the vascular function of the heart, brain, blood pressure and arteries by an additional 6.2% in a dose-dependent fashion. This conference also showed that in eight separate studies with more than 257,000 participants, that there was a 26% reduction in the risk of strokes among those people who consumed more than 5 portions of fruits and vegetables per day. This study was reported in the *Journal of Nutrition*, and involved 221,000 men and women (*Family Practice News* – January 15, 2009).

The nutrients in fruits and vegetables, such as dietary fiber and antioxidants, are associated with a lower risk of heart disease, but few studies have examined their relationship to the risk for stroke. This study, reported in the *Journal of the American Medical Association,* described the association between fruit and vegetable intake and ischemic stroke in over 75,000 woman enrolled in the Nurses' Health Study and 38,000 men in the health professional follow-up study. Everyone in this particular study had no history of cardiovascular disease, stroke, cancer, diabetes, or high cholesterol. During the follow-up period, which included fourteen years for women and eight years for men, each increment of one serving of fruit or vegetables per day was associated with a 7% reduction for risk of ischemic stroke in women, and a 4% reduction in men. This would translate into a *35% reduction in stroke for women* who ate five servings daily of fruit and vegetables. This study showed that there was no further reduction in the risk of stroke above 5-6 servings of fruit and vegetables per day. The consumption of a variety of vegetables and fruits, such as cruciferous vegetables (examples: broccoli and cabbage), green, leafy vegetables, citrus fruits or vitamin C-rich fruits and vegetables resulted in the largest decrease in risk. Pretty impressive results by just following your high-fiber diet of fruits and veggies.

In a recent study in the *American Journal of Epidemiology,* women on a high-fiber diet showed a significantly reduced risk from coronary heart disease and death from all causes. This study reviewed dietary data from the Scottish Heart Study on approximately 12,000 women and men, 40–59 years of age. Those people with a high intake of fiber had the greatest reduced risk of mortality from all causes, including coronary heart disease. These results suggest that the current public health drive to increase the nutrient and fiber intake to at least five portions of fruit and vegetables a day should have beneficial effects on all causes of mortality. This study also showed that consuming high levels of fiber and antioxidants was associated with significantly lower rates of coronary heart disease and all types of mortality.

TEN TIPS TO ADD LOTS OF FIBER TO YOUR DIET

1. **Drink 6-8 glasses of water daily.** Fiber can absorb many times its own weight of water, providing bulk to the diet and a subsequent feeling of fullness. A high fiber diet requires that you drink lots of water, so that the fiber can absorb much of the water and create bulk in the intestines, which makes you feel full, before you've had a chance to eat too much.

2. **Eat high-fiber whole grain cereals for breakfast**, preferably those with 5 or more grams of fiber per serving. You can beef up the fiber

content of cereals by adding 1½ Tbs. of unprocessed bran or wheat germ, if necessary. Each level teaspoon contains two grams of dietary fiber. Either may be sprinkled on cereal or other foods, or it may be mixed in with orange or tomato juice to improve its taste. Be careful of so-called, "healthy granola cereals," many of which have a high saturated fat content and little fiber. Some granola cereals; however, are low in fat and high in fiber. Always check the ingredients label.

3. **Breads must have the word "whole"** as the first listed ingredient on the package; otherwise it's not a true whole-grain product, no matter how the bread is labeled. Substitute whole grain bread (stone ground or whole wheat) or fiber enriched bread and bran instead of white refined breads. Whole grain and fiber-enriched breads have more than double the fiber content of white bread.

4. **Use whole grain flour or soy flour** instead of refined white flour. Eat whole grain pastas in place of regular pasta. Select bran and whole grain cereals, brown long grain rice, and whole grain noodles.

5. **Eat fresh fruit with skin**, rather than fruit juices, which have little or no fiber content. Increase fruits (apples, oranges, pears, bananas, strawberries, blueberries, plums, pitted dried prunes, peaches and cherries).

6. **Consume more vegetables**, legumes and salads (without the dressing, of course, unless you use a little olive oil and vinegar). Include carrots, celery, cabbage, peas, broccoli, brussels sprouts, lentils, potatoes with skin, dried beans and baked beans (without sugar or bacon). Add other garden vegetables such as green beans, lettuce, onions, corn, peas, tomatoes, and spinach.

7. **Add bran**, wheat germ, nuts, seeds, legumes, beans or grits to soups (not creamed), yogurt or casseroles. Unprocessed bran and wheat germ are dry bran/wheat powders, which are convenient, high dietary fibers.

8. **Snack foods** should include dried fruits including pitted prunes, nuts, seeds, bran cereals, snack bars (high-fiber, low fat), rice cakes, popcorn, celery and carrot sticks.

9. **Popcorn** is an excellent high-fiber, low-fat, low-calorie snack. Use non- or low-fat varieties. Without the added salt, oil, and butter, popcorn is probably one of the best diet snacks available. It is low in calories and cholesterol, and high in fiber. It consequently fills you up without adding extra calories and provides 2 grams of fiber per 1½ cups. One cup of popcorn contains only 25 calories. The electric hot-air popper is, by far, the most efficient way to prepare popcorn. Since it uses no oil, there are no added fats, and there is no cleanup necessary. These hot-air poppers can produce great quantities of popcorn in a relatively short period of time. This electric appliance is a must for your low-cholesterol, high-fiber walking diet. Most microwaveable popcorns contain considerable fat; however, several newer products are available in low-fat varieties. Always check the label.

10. **Start adding fiber slowly** to your diet to avoid cramping, bloating, or gas. Make small additions of fiber-rich foods over a period of four to six weeks. If you find that a particular high-fiber food causes cramping or bloating, discontinue eating it and try another type of high-fiber food. Continue to increase your daily fiber intake until you reach 40 grams of fiber a day for good health and weight reduction. Remember, it's very important to drink more fluids as you increase your fiber intake. You should drink between 6-8 glasses of water daily. Fiber can absorb many times its own weight. This provides excess bulk to the diet, which makes you feel full so that you cut down on the total number of calories that you consume daily. This excess bulk formed by fiber and water also helps to keep your intestinal tract healthy. Philly's Fit-Step Walking Diet adds the necessary fiber to your diet, which helps you lose weight quickly, stay healthy, and live longer.

2013 CURRENT DIETARY GUIDELINES

According to large scale studies reported in 2013 by The American Heart Association and The American College of Cardiology, they recommended new guidelines on healthier dietary changes in order to reduce the incidence of cardiovascular risk.

1. These guidelines recommend a dietary pattern that emphasizes fruits and vegetables, whole grains, legumes, fish, white meat poultry, nuts and vegetable oils such as olive oil. They also recommend restricted consumption of saturated and trans fats especially red meat and processed meat, and sugar and sodium.

2. Eating three or more portions of fruits and veggies daily reduced the risk of coronary artery disease, hypertension, strokes, and the degenerative diseases of aging, including some forms of cancer.

3. This study determined a positive association between the consumption of red meat and processed meat with a high mortality from cardiovascular disease and cancer. Daily consumption of red meat at an average 5.6 oz. or more was independently associated with a 14% higher risk of all causes of mortality. People who ate an average of 5.6 oz. or more daily of processed meats had a 44% greater risk of all causes of mortality. These studies concluded that low meat consumption was associated with increased longevity.

4. The increased consumption of nuts was associated with a stepwise reduction in all causes of mortality. People who consumed nuts less than once a week had a 7% reduction in the risk of total mortality, compared with those who didn't eat nuts. People who ate nuts once per week had an 11% reduction in risk; those who ate nuts 2-4 times per week had a 13% reduction in risk; those who ate nuts 5 or 6 times per week had a 15% reduction in risk; and people who ate nuts seven or more times per week had a 20% reduction in the risk of all causes of mortality.

Jancin, B., *Family Practice News*, March 1, 2014, Vol.44, No. 4, pp 22-25.

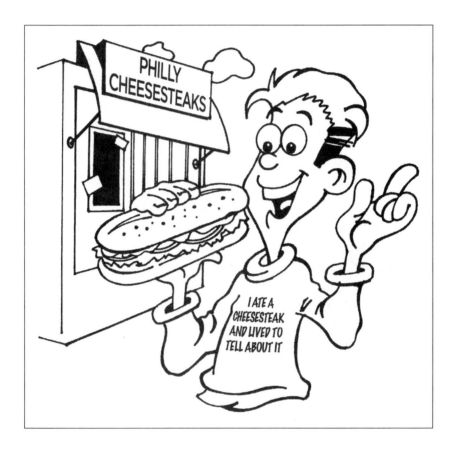

EAT A PHILLY CHEESESTEAK

A ccording to *Men's Fitness Magazine*, Philadelphia is among "America's Fattest Cities." By its very nature, Philadelphia is a fat city, since we are known for our cheesesteaks, hoagies or submarines, scrapple, pork sausage, bacon, pulled-pork sandwiches, hotdogs, chicken wings, beer, and chips. Perhaps if the good citizens of Philadelphia would start a simple exercise program like walking, they would be able to lose weight, shape up, look and feel better and certainly live longer. People from Philadelphia and other "Fat Cities" have to realize that in addition to a healthy diet, a walking program has many health, fitness and longevity benefits that can counteract their poor eating habits.

Like many American Cities, Philadelphia is just starting to make an effort to slim down. There are lots of new restaurants and markets that specialize in healthy, nutritious foods. For example, the Reading Terminal Market in Center City Philadelphia, and the Italian Market in South Philly has an array of healthy foods including fresh fruits and vegetables, fish, and low fat meats. These markets also carry numerous food products that are free of chemicals, pesticides and hormones. In addition, there are many health food stores and markets throughout the city that specialize in an assortment of healthy food products.

Once the people of the "City of Brotherly Love" realize that by limiting their cheesesteaks and other fatty foods and increasing their walking habits, Philadelphia will begin to lose its "fat city" status. Philadelphians are in the early stages of a diet and exercise revolution. Philadelphia is an excellent aerobic walking city. The streets were originally designed by William Penn and laid out in a grid- like pattern of walking paths through historical, commercial and residential streets. You'll find excellent walking tours and walking paths in the following books:

1. Colimore, Edward. *The Philadelphia Inquirer's Walking Tours of Historic Philadelphia.* Philadelphia: Camino Books, 2007.

2. ----------. *Insight City Guide: Philadelphia.* Ed. John Gattuso. Long Island City: Langenscheidt Publishers, 2007.

3. Varr, Richard. *Eyewitness Travel: Philadelphia and the Pennsylvania Dutch Country.* New York: DK Publishing, Inc., 2007

Other towns and cities throughout the United States have excellent walking paths and tours as well. You can contact your own city's libraries, bookstores and information centers for details.

HOW TO EAT A PHILLY CHEESESTEAK & LIVE TO TELL THE TALE

You must realize that a single Philly Cheesesteak contains more saturated fat than most people consume in two or three days. But never fear, I'll show you how you can safely eat one of one of our delicious Philly Cheesesteaks without actually doubling your cholesterol level and live to tell the tale.

• First of all, remove approximately one-half of the meat in the sandwich. Even the amount of meat remaining will be tremendous.

• Secondly, scoop out your roll, and then put the meat back in.

• Use provolone cheese instead of cheese whiz.

• Go light on the fried onions and skip the sauce.

• Add lettuce and tomato.

Enjoy! You'll actually be eating a delicious Philly cheesesteak with approximately one-third the calories and one-third the amount of saturated fat which is contained in a regular Philly cheesesteak. A regular cheesesteak actually contains approximately 1,600 calories and approximately 38 grams of saturated fat. Be very afraid!

DIETARY FAT REALLY MAKES YOU FAT!

It's very difficult to imagine how many fat calories you consume each day. It's important to be able to find the fat in your diet and eliminate it. Everyone knows that there's fat in meat, sausage, bacon, lunchmeats, eggs, butter, ice cream, milk, and cheese. But not everyone realizes that there's a considerable amount of fat in donuts, cakes, pies, muffins, margarine, mayonnaise, chicken and tuna salad, coffee creamers, yogurt, cream cheese and cottage cheese. Also, it's important to remember that there are 9 calories in each gram of fat we eat, compared to 4 calories in each gram of protein or carbohydrate that we consume. The more fat calories you consume, the more fat will be stored in your body, and the more weight you will gain. Dietary fat just fills up your fat cells because hardly any of the fat calories (only five out of 1,000) are used for digestion and are therefore not burned up. In other words fat not only is unhealthy, but it actually makes you fat.

Your body metabolizes fats and carbohydrates together in a set ratio governed genetically by your individual body's metabolism. When you restrict the number of fat calories that you consume, then your body's metabolism automatically controls the amount of refined carbohydrate calories that you actually eat. By restricting the fat calories eaten *you crave fewer refined carbohydrates in your diet.* The combination of less fat eaten combined with less refined carbohydrates craved, makes it next to impossible for you to put on excess weight. So when you eat less fat you're less likely to get fat. Sounds simple? It is! That's one of the ways that the Philly Fit-Step Walking Diet works.

The most important part of any successful diet is starting it. Once you've made up your mind to begin your diet, you're half way there. The Fit-Step Walking Diet consists of eating no more than 40 Grams of Fat and no less than 40 Grams Fiber. This diet is very easy to follow and you see results quickly. When this diet is combined with walking for 40 minutes (or 20 minutes twice daily), six days per week and walking with hand-held weights, 2 or 3 days per week, you have the perfect combination of a double blast of calorie burning. First you burn calories by the actual aerobic exercise of walking. Secondly, you burn additional calories by building muscle tissue with the strength training exercise of walking with weights. *Philly's Fit-Step Walking Diet is the best step for permanent weight-loss and physical fitness!*

HEART DISEASE CAUSED BY EXCESS DIETARY FAT

When you consume excess amounts of saturated fats, the fat that accumulates has to go someplace. You can see what's happening on the outside of you. Now, let's take a look at the inside. Fat infiltrates the liver and other organs. Fat compresses the heart and decreases the blood supply to the rest of the body's organs, tissues and cells. Along with all of this, extra heavy people, and even moderately overweight persons, are putting an extra burden on their backs and legs (the weight bearing joints), which causes or increases arthritic problems. Complications following surgery occur more frequently in obese people. Wounds don't heal as well or as fast. And, overweight people can't tolerate anesthesia as well as people of normal weight, usually because of breathing problems.

In a study just released by the National Heart, Lung and Blood Institute in Bethesda, Maryland, obesity has now been listed as a major independent risk factor for heart disease. What's so new about that? Everyone knows that being overweight contributes to heart disease. That's just it; up until now obesity was just a contributing factor in heart disease because of its relationship with high blood pressure and high cholesterol. Now it has gained its own independent rating as causing heart disease all by itself. This study, consisting of 5,000 women and men, was followed for 26 years. The risk of developing heart disease was more pronounced in people who gained most of their excess weight after the age of 25. In this study, obesity ranked third in men and fourth in women in predicting coronary heart disease. Only high blood pressure, cholesterol, and age were ranked ahead of obesity, with cigarette smoking a close fourth in predicting heart disease. One important point made in this extensive study was: losing a moderate amount of weight lessened the risk of developing heart disease.

According to the American Heart Association, more than 41 million Americans have one or more forms of heart or blood vessel disease. **Heart attacks** claimed 685,000 lives in 2010 and 60 percent of all deaths come from cardiovascular disease. The Heart Association estimated that as many as one million Americans will have a heart attack this year and more than one-third of them will die.

Strokes were listed as the second leading cause of death in cardiovascular disease, which claimed 210,000 lives in 2010. They estimated that 2.1 million Americans are survivors of stroke. One in every four adults or 35 million Americans suffer from **high blood pressure**. In 2010, over 295,000 people died from the complications of high blood pressure.

It has recently been discovered that red meat in addition to its excess content of saturated fat, contains a molecule called *Carnitine* , which when digested by the bacteria in your intestine actually speeds up the process of hardening of the arteries in the heart, brain and peripheral blood vessels. Here's another really good reason to stay away from red meat.

TYPES OF FATS

I. SATURATED FAT

Saturated fat is present in all products of animal origin: meat, fish, fowl, eggs, butter, milk, cream and cheese. Saturated fats are also found in some vegetable products, which are usually solid or semi-solid at room temperature. They include shortenings and table spreads which have been changed from liquid fats (usually cottonseed and soybean oils) into solids by a process called hydrogenation. This process makes the products more suitable for table use and prevents them from becoming rancid. However, this process converts polyunsaturated fats into saturated fats. Other saturated fats in the vegetable kingdom include cocoa butter, palm oil and coconut oil. Most people are unaware of the fact that they consume significant amounts of coconut and palm oil. It is used commercially in a wide variety of processed foods, baked goods and deep-fat fried products.

Saturated fats are dangerous because they can increase the amount of cholesterol in the blood. These fats can raise the level of blood cholesterol as much as, if not more than, the actual consumption of dietary cholesterol products. These fats can also interfere with brain function and can actually cause damage to the brain cells by interfering with the brain's circulation. This can lead to memory loss, difficulty concentrating, and confusion and may even accelerate Alzheimer's disease. These fats also raise your bad LDL cholesterol and lower your good HDL cholesterol.

II. UNSATURATED FATS

1. **Monounsaturated fats** (neutral fats) may actually help to increase the good HDL cholesterol level, and, therefore, they have been found to be **cardio-protective**. These fats contain **omega-3 fatty acids** which are extremely important in decreasing your risk of heart disease, degenerative diseases of aging, and certain forms of cancer. These fats are usually liquid at room temperature and tend to harden or cloud when refrigerated. They are the primary fats found in olive oil, canola oil, peanut oil, most nuts and seeds, olives, avocados and some whole grain products. You should cook with **monounsaturated oils** such as olive oil, canola oil, or peanut oil. And you should eat monounsaturated foods such as soybeans, seeds, nuts, olives, and avocados. These are the best of all of the fats and are considered to be heart-protective.

2. **Polyunsaturated fats** (essential fatty acids) are always of vegetable origin and are liquid oils. Safflower oil is the highest in polyunsaturates of all oils. Sunflower oil is second, followed by corn oil, sesame seed oil, soybean oil, cottonseed oil, walnut oil and linseed oil. Polyunsaturated fats in limited amounts may help to lower the bad LDL cholesterol level by assisting the body to eliminate excessive amounts of newly manufactured cholesterol. It is essential that you substitute monounsaturated and polyunsaturated fats for saturated fats to maximize their cholesterol-lowering effect. It is

interesting to note that we can manufacture saturated fat and most monounsaturated fats in our bodies. Polyunsaturated fats, however, must be obtained from the diet and are, therefore, called **omega -6 essential fatty acids**. These can be considered bad fats when excessive amounts are consumed, since they can set up chronic inflammation in brain tissue, which could lead to brain damage, strokes and degenerative brain diseases like Alzheimer's disease. Therefore, polyunsaturated oils should be limited to 1½ tsp. daily. Otherwise these are considered to be **good fats in moderation**.

3. **Trans-fats** are fats that are formed when hydrogen atoms are added to oils containing mono or polyunsaturated fats. The hydrogenation process converts liquid oils into a more solid form. They then become hydrogenated (solid) or partially hydrogenated (semi-solid) oils and are **very bad fats**. Trans fat was originally put into the food supply in response to consumer's concerns about the health effects of animal fats. Unfortunately, these trans fats were actually found to me more dangerous than saturated animal fats. They can increase your risk of heart disease by raising your bad LDL cholesterol and decreasing your good HDL cholesterol. Since labeling began in 2010, consumption of trans fat is down considerably. The CDC tracked grocery items from 2007 through 2012, and found a 49% decrease in trans fats present in the foods.

They also have been reported to release a chemical called **Tumor Necrosis Factor**, which can cause inflammation in the body, thus increasing the risk for heart attacks, diabetes, high blood pressure and cancer. They are found in cooking oils, shortening, margarine many processed and baked foods, cookies, crackers, snack foods, and non-dairy creamers. Always check food labels for hydrogenated or partially hydrogenated oils, which are actually trans-fats.

Avoid any and all foods that have hydrogenated or partially hydrogenated oils as ingredients listed on the label. Even if the product states that the amount of Trans-fats is 0, and they list hydrogenated and partially hydrogenated oils on the label, and then avoid this product since their labeling is misleading.

HOW TRANS FATS ADD POUNDS TO YOUR WEIGHT

1. Ordinarily, when carbohydrates are eaten they are absorbed from the intestinal tract and converted to glucose in the blood stream. This glucose is absorbed into the body's cells for the production of energy and some of it is stored in the liver and muscles as a form of stored energy called **glycogen**. Glycogen remains in the liver and muscles for future use in the production of energy. When fats are consumed, however, some of them are converted into fatty acids in the blood stream. Fatty acids are readily incorporated into muscle and fat cells throughout the body. Normally fatty acids in muscle cells can be used by the muscle cell membranes for the production of energy by converting fatty acids into glucose. These fatty acids help the muscle cells absorb and utilize blood glucose for the production of energy.

2. Trans fats, however, are absorbed into the muscle cell membrane and negatively affect the muscle cell's ability to absorb glucose from the blood stream and its ability to convert it into a useful form of energy. When these active muscle cells can not absorb and metabolize glucose, blood sugar levels spike and subsequently cause spikes in blood insulin levels. These increased levels of insulin causes fat to be stored in the body's fat cells since they can not get inside the metabolically active muscle cells. This excess accumulation of fat inside the body's fat cells results in rapid weight gain and subsequent obesity, especially if the consumption of Trans fats continues.

3. Trans fats can block the production of the appetite suppressant hormone and mood relaxing hormone such as serotonin, dopamine and nor-epinephrine. These toxic fats accomplish this nefarious deed by causing the cells in your brain to become inflamed. This inflammatory process results in an increased appetite and food craving and the subsequent increase in the consumption of excess calories. This toxic process also contributes to anxiety and insomnia. People tend to eat more bad

carbs when they can not fall asleep causing additional fat to be stored in your body's fat cells.

4. Trans fats also cause you to gain more belly fat by redistributing stored fatty acids from various locations throughout the body and sending them into the abdominal fat cells. This increase in belly fat is thought to be due to the fact while trans fats cause a toxic reaction in the body's fat cells, causing them to discharge particles of fat globules into the blood stream and relocating these fat globules into the abdominal area (the omentum which is a curtain of fat cells lining the abdominal intestinal organs). This omentum is located in the middle of the body and in the direct path of these traveling fat globules. Since there are so many fat cells located in the omentum, it is like a large fish net that catches all of these migrating fat cells and stores them as abdominal fat.

5. There are many foods and compounds which help to eliminate trans fats from the body. These include the omega-3 fatty acids which are present in fish oils and flaxseeds. These healthy fatty acids help to produce a compound called cholecystokinin which helps to decrease hunger and helps to counteract the adverse effects of fatty acids on the intestinal tract and liver. Also, citrus foods such as oranges, limes and lemons contain the antioxidant vitamin C, which helps to eliminate free radicals which occur from the ingestion of fatty acids. Vegetables such as brussels sprouts, broccoli, cabbage and cauliflower are known as cruciferous vegetables. They contain compounds called *sulforaphane* and *indole-3 carbinol* which help to eliminate trans fats from the intestinal tract and help the liver's ability to convert these Trans fats into water soluble components which can be easily eliminated by the intestinal tract. Several fruits contain phytochemicals called *anthocyanins* which are found in papaya, guava, kiwi and cranberries. These rich and powerful phytochemicals can cause the elimination of trans fats from the body, particularly if these fruits are consumed in blended drinks. The anthocyanin rich fruits

that are contained in blended fruit juices can combine with the trans fats and eliminate them from the intestinal tract.

SAY NO-NO TO YO-YO DIETS

The Framingham Heart Study, which has followed more than 5,000 people for almost 40 years, recently indicated a health hazard for chronic dieters. People who lost 10% of their body weight had an almost 20% reduction in the incidence of heart disease. So what's the problem? These same dieters, who gained back the 10% of their body weight, raised their heart disease risk by almost 30%. So if you weigh 160 lbs. and lost 10% or 16 lbs., you decreased your heart disease risk by 20%. But if you gained back those 16 lbs., you increased your risk of heart attack by 30%, an overall net gain of 10% and you still weigh the same 160 lbs. So you're actually back where you started. It seems like a waste of time and effort on your part. How many times have you heard the old saying that "I've lost enough weight over the years to equal two or three whole persons and I've gained every bit of it back?" Yo-yo dieting or weight-cycling makes it harder to permanently lose weight and is much more dangerous to your health.

1. The **weight-loss/weight-gain cycle** actually increases your desire for fatty foods. Animal research studies at Yale University showed that rats that had lost weight rapidly on low-calorie diets always chose more fat in their diets when given a choice between fat, protein, and carbohydrates. These rats always put on more weight than when they started and in a much shorter time than it had taken them to lose the weight.

2. **Yo-yo dieters increase the ratio of body fat** to lean body tissue with repeated bouts of weight gain and weight loss. People who lose weight rapidly on a low carbohydrate-high protein diet can lose a significant amount of muscle tissue. If the weight is regained again, they usually regain more fat and less muscle because it is easier for the body to gain fat than it is to rebuild muscle tissue.

3. **Body fat gets redistributed in the abdomen from the thighs, buttocks and hips** after weight cycling. Medical research has

definitely shown that fat deposits above the waist increases the risk of heart disease and diabetes, not to mention an unsightly paunch.

4. When you lose weight by cutting calories, your **basal metabolic rate (BMR)** goes down, because it is the body's defense mechanism against starvation. The body can't tell the difference between starvation and low calorie dieting; consequently, your body is trying to conserve energy by burning fewer calories. This is the reason it becomes harder to lose weight after a week or two, even though you are eating exactly the same amount of calories as you did when you first started your diet. This slow-down in the basal metabolic rate (BMR) persists even after the diet is over and accounts for the rapid-rebound, excessive weight gain that always happens to the dieter when she goes off her diet. This slow-down in metabolic rate can occur even after a single attempt at dieting. However, the repeated effects of weight-cycling diets can affect the basal metabolic rate (BMR) much more, making additional weight-loss almost impossible and rebound weight gain almost inevitable. The yo-yo dieter is often heard to say —"I'm heavier now than I was before I started this damn diet."

5. An enzyme called **lipoprotein lipase (LPL)** becomes more active when you cut calories. This enzyme controls the amount of fat that is stored in your body's fat cells. Dieting, therefore, makes the body more efficient at storing fat, which is exactly the opposite of what a dieter wants. As you reduce your calorie intake, the enzyme LPL starts to activate the fat-storing process. This is another defense mechanism that the body uses to prevent starvation. Remember, the enzyme LPL doesn't know that you are dieting; it thinks that you are actually starving.

6. Women and men dieters who've lost a substantial amount of weight were compared to a group of normal weight people. After they lost weight, the previously obese individuals needed surprisingly fewer calories to maintain their weight than the normal-weight women. In this study, obese people who lost weight needed only 2000 calories a day to maintain their weight (125 lbs.) compared

to 2300 calories per day to maintain the exact same weight (125 lbs.) by normal-weight people. Who said dieting was fair?

7. Chronic dieters who exhibited repeated cycles of weight gain and weight loss showed an increased risk of sudden death from heart attacks, according to a recent medical report, which followed 1500 women over a period of 25 years who had engaged in cyclic-dieting.

SAY YES-YES TO WALKING

We know that losing weight lowers blood pressure, reduces the risk of heart disease, lowers blood cholesterol and triglycerides and increases the HDL ("good" cholesterol). But dieting alone is not the best way to lose and maintain weight. The following is a list of the reasons why **walking** is the only safe and effective method to lose and maintain your ideal body weight:

1. **Exercise**, **particularly walking**, is the real answer to preventing the weight loss/weight-gain cycle from occurring. Walking makes it less likely you'll gain the weight back again because you lose more fat and less muscle tissue with exercise. Also, walking prevents the slow-down in basal metabolic rate that always occurs with a yo-yo diet. In fact, walking slightly **increases the BMR,** which helps to burn calories at a faster rate. Walking also **reduces the production of the enzyme lipoprotein lipase (LPL)**, which in turn decreases the amount of fat stored in the fat cells.

2. Walking also regulates the brain's appetite controller, the **appestat**. The more you walk, the more you decrease the appestat's hunger mechanism. Inactivity, on the other hand, stimulates the appetite control mechanism to make you hungry.

3. Walking, by increasing the aerobic metabolism of the body, **redirects the stomach's blood supply** to the exercising muscles, which in turn decreases your appetite.

4. And finally, walking for 40 minutes six days per week or 20 minutes twice daily encourages the body to *burn fat rather than*

carbohydrates. This enables the body's blood sugar to stay at a relatively constant normal level. When the brain's blood sugar is normal we are not hungry. Both strenuous exercise and low-calorie dieting, however, burn carbohydrates rather than fats, causing a sharp drop in the blood sugar. When the brain's blood sugar drops as it does in dieting or strenuous exercises, then we feel hungry in order to counteract this low blood sugar. The high fiber content of the Philly Fit -Step Diet also controls the body's appetite center, making overeating high-fat calories next to impossible.

Boost Your Fat-Burning Metabolism

1. You will burn more calories if you *eat small, frequent meals* or snack every three to four hours. Eating small, frequent meals help keep the body's **insulin level** more even, which makes it less likely you will store fat. If you go for a long period between large meals, your insulin levels spike, which makes it more likely you will store the extra calories and sugar as fat. This is because sporadic surges in insulin levels cause more sugar to be stored in your body's cells as fat, rather than being used as a source of fuel to produce energy.

2. People, who eat a skimpy breakfast or no breakfast at all and very little lunch, save up all of their calories for a big meal at dinner. This is probably the worst way to burn fat and the best way to store fat because of the inefficient utilization of glucose as a fuel. Instead *glucose gets turned into fat stores* in the body's cells.

3. If you eat every few hours you will have more energy because sugar will be used efficiently as **fuel to produce energy**. On the other hand, if you eat infrequently or wait until you are famished, then you will be fatigued because the sugar will not be able to be used as fuel efficiently, and energy production will go down.

   a. Your brain needs **fuel to produce energy** to enable you to think clearly, concentrate, and to work efficiently. Also your body needs fuel to help you exercise for longer periods of time, and to move faster and more efficiently. This steady supply of fuel can only be accomplished by a steady supply of glucose being utilized to produce the energy required for proper brain and body function.

    b. So the formula is: small frequent, high fiber, lean protein, complex carbohydrate meals = steady level of insulin = constant supply of glucose = production of energy to boost body and mind functions.

4. It is important to have **a snack** (piece of fruit or a small amount of whole grain cereal or a slice of whole grain bread) before your walking exercise workout (with or without weights), in order to increase your production of energy. Exercise stabilizes insulin and glucose levels, so that energy production is maximized. The combination of exercise and a small helpful snack improves your energy level.

5. On Philly's Fit-Step Walking Diet, the addition of a moderate amount of **lean protein** (very lean meats, white meat of chicken or turkey, fish, non-fat dairy products (including cheeses, milk, yogurt, soy and egg whites), whole grains and bran, nuts and seeds, all contribute to burning fat calories and boosting energy. Protein suppresses your appetite and produces the necessary fuel for the production of energy for all of your body's needs. Protein is made up of amino acids, which are essential for your cells' metabolism and for the repair and maintenance of all of your body's cells.

6. Several recent research studies have confirmed that people, who consume two to three servings of **calcium containing foods** such as milk, cheese, or yogurt daily, lost considerably more weight than those individuals who just reduced their calorie intake, while consuming very little in the way of dairy products. This is true of people who consume calcium-containing foods as opposed to taking calcium supplements, which can cause a build-up of harmful plaque in the arteries. This adverse effect seems to be offset if you consume adequate amounts of Vitamin D along with calcium supplements.

High calcium diets have been proven to inhibit the production of a certain calcium-regulating hormone, so that the amount of calcium and fat stored in the body's cells actually decreases. This actually causes you to store less fat, and ultimately lose more weight. On the other hand, it has been shown that low calcium diets actually increase this calcium-regulating hormone, which causes both calcium and fat to be stored in the body's cells and ultimately causes weight to be gained.

This calcium-regulating hormone works in conjunction with the protein found in dairy products to burn fat more efficiently and more quickly, which is another reason dairy products help you to lose weight. Research studies have also shown that low fat dairy products have the same ability to limit fat storage and burn fat calories, as does whole milk dairy products. So non-fat milk, yogurt, and low-fat cheeses are ideal for a weight reduction program.

Newer research has even shown that people burn more fat in their abdominal region (waist circumference), and subsequently lose more inches by combining two to three low-fat dairy products a day with a high fiber, low fat diet. This reduction in abdominal fat can help to decrease the risk of diabetes, high blood pressure, heart disease, and a condition known as the metabolic syndrome (high blood pressure, diabetes, obesity, coronary artery disease). For people who are lactose intolerant, lactose-free milk and yogurt work just as well.

METABOLIC SYNDROME: FIT OR FAT?

In a recent study reported at the Third World Congress in 2012, it was shown that a patient's fitness level is as important as obesity in the development of the metabolic syndrome, as well as in all causes of mortality. This was due in part to a condition known as the insulin resistance syndrome, which results from the patient's inability to process and utilize insulin effectively.

People with low levels of cardiovascular and cardio respiratory fitness and those with low levels of muscular strength were prone to develop the metabolic syndrome to a greater degree than those patients who were just obese. The metabolic syndrome is defined as a condition that is composed of diabetes, high blood pressure, obesity, high lipids, and cardiovascular disease. It has been previously thought that obesity was the major factor in the development of the metabolic syndrome; however, it has been recently discovered that low levels of fitness also contribute to the development of this syndrome.

Patients with moderate to high levels of cardiovascular fitness were found to be significantly less likely to develop the metabolic syndrome than were those individuals with low fitness levels. This study suggested that a patient's low level of fitness may be more important than his/her obesity in determining his/her risk for developing the metabolic syndrome. Improved muscular strength was shown to decrease an individual's likelihood of developing the metabolic syndrome, possibly because of the muscles ability to process insulin and sugar more effectively.

METABOLIC SYNDROME WARNING SIGNS

1. Waist size greater than 36 inches for women and 42 inches for men

2. Blood pressure over 140/90

3. HDL cholesterol less than 50 in women and less than 40 in men

4. LDL cholesterol more than 110 in either men or women

5. Cholesterol levels over 220

6. Triglyceride levels over 180

MELT BELLY FAT

Refined carbohydrates that we eat are gradually absorbed into the blood stream, which causes a sudden spike in insulin production. This excess amount of insulin in our blood causes these digested refined carbohydrates to head straight into our fat cells, particularly our belly fat cells, since the abdominal or belly fat cells are the closest to the digestive tract and contain the most concentrated amounts of fat cells in the entire body. Once the excess insulin has done its work by lowering the blood sugar and packing fat into the fat cells of the abdomen, the low blood sugar which results, causes another round of carbohydrate cravings. It is like a "lose-lose combination."

As we age, we crave more carbohydrates, and the more carbs we eat, the more calories become stored as fat in our abdomen. Due to certain hormonal changes which regular our digestive system, we become less able to burn carbs for fuel, thus making carbs more likely to become stored as fat in the body, particularly in the abdomen. This actually becomes a vicious cycle since the more carbs we store as belly fat, the more carbohydrates we crave in our diet. Stored abdominal fat suppresses the formation of fat-burning hormones such as *leptin* which helps to keep blood sugars steady. Consequently, the more abdominal fat that you store makes it easier for you to gain more weight.

If you can lose abdominal fat, then you will diminish carbohydrate cravings and subsequently lose the unwanted belly fat. By eating high fiber foods you can actually block the absorption of refined carbohydrates and starches. This is accomplished by the increased fiber foods preventing the absorption of these refined carbohydrates by forming a web or net of fibers which encircles or tangles up these starches and carries them out of the digestive tract, almost completely intact and undigested. By blocking most of the absorption of these refined starches, less sugar and insulin are present in the blood stream, which subsequently results in fewer cravings for carbohydrates. Less craving for carbs results in more belly fat than being burned and more weight being loss, particularly around the abdomen.

Since high fiber foods, particularly beans (white, kidney, fava and pinto beans) contain an enzyme-blocking compound which blocks pancreatic enzymes (amylase and lipase) from breaking down refined starches. By inhibiting these enzymes from absorbing refined carbohydrates, your digestive tract bypasses absorption of these starches and transports them out of your digestive tract as though they were never totally digested. This results in a much slower rise in blood sugar, which in turns does not cause a spike in insulin production and consequently reduces your craving for carbohydrates.

BELLY FAT MELTING TIPS

THE FIBER-MINERAL COMBO—foods that contain both fiber and the mineral magnesium help to decrease the risk of developing the so-called **metabolic syndrome**. This syndrome consists of high blood pressure, diabetes, high blood fats, particularly triglycerides, insulin resistance, obesity and a tendency to accumulate excess amounts of abdominal fat. The combination of magnesium and fiber prevents sudden spikes in blood sugar and blood insulin levels that cause excess amounts of fat to become stored in your body's abdominal fat cells. Foods rich in magnesium include peas, beans (Lima and kidney beans), avocados, spinach, broccoli, whole grains, wheat germ, brown rice, sweet potatoes with skin and many fruits.

LOW-FAT DAIRY PRODUCTS (CHEESE, MILK, YOGURT)—these low-fat dairy products suppress the hormone Calcitrol that causes fat to be stored in your abdominal fat cells. These low-fat dairy products also reduce the risk of developing the metabolic syndrome by up to 50%. Also, the combination of calcium and protein in these daily products combine to burn additional calories and help in weight-loss.

ELIMINATE TRANS FATS—Trans fats can almost double your risk of developing the metabolic syndrome. These fats are either hydrogenated or partially hydrogenated oils that are found in margarine, fast and frozen foods, baked goods, non-dairy creamers and most packaged and processed foods. These fats can raise your blood pressure and increase your blood sugar, and therefore, block your arteries with cholesterol deposits. Recent research has shown that for every 3 to 5% increase in the consumption of Trans fats, results in a 2 pound weight gain every four to six weeks, particularly around the abdominal wall.

AVOID STRESS—You can avoid stress by meditating, walking, doing yoga, or any activity that you find calming. Stress unfortunately causes the body to produce the stress hormone cortisol that can increase your blood fats, particularly the triglycerides, and also increases your blood pressure and blood sugar. This deadly combination increases your risk of developing insulin resistance, which subsequently produces more belly fat, and thus, increases the risk of developing the metabolic syndrome. Recent studies have shown that reducing cortisol production by engaging in calming activities and exercise helps to prevent the development of the metabolic syndrome with all of its attendant hazards including excess storage of belly fat.

FOLLOW THE MEDITERRANEAN DIET—The Mediterranean diet consists primarily of fruits, vegetables, whole grains, nuts, olive oil, and fish and small amounts of lean meats and poultry. This diet can actually reduce the risk of developing the metabolic syndrome by up to 50%. The diet improves blood sugar and insulin control and reduces blood pressure simply by increasing the intake of plant foods. The monounsaturated heart-healthy olive oil helps to decrease blood pressure, blood sugar, obesity, blood fats, coronary artery disease, cancer and degenerative diseases. This diet increases the level of good HDL cholesterol by more than 30% which acts to clear out cholesterol deposits in blocked arteries, thus decreasing the risk of heart attacks and strokes

FAT-FIGHTING FACTS

1. **Don't skip breakfast.** Studies have proved that people who eat a healthy breakfast every day are the most successful dieters. Healthy breakfasts of whole-grain, high-fiber cereal topped with fruit and skim milk is a great way to start the day, or an egg fried in a small amount of olive oil on a slice of toasted whole-wheat bread makes a great lean protein start for your day. A slice of whole-wheat bread topped with a Tbs. of all-fruit jelly and/ or peanut butter is an appetite-satisfying breakfast. People who regularly eat a healthy breakfast don't get hungry for midmorning snacks of doughnuts or muffins. Your body's appetite control mechanism stays in check for long periods of time, without any spikes in blood sugar or blood insulin levels. And besides, a nutritious breakfast causes your body to burn fat more efficiently and starts your diet-day off perfectly.

2. **Sneak in the veggies and the fruits.** Most people don't get their three servings each of fruits and vegetables daily. The way to sneak in your daily allotment of fruits and vegetables is to add them to most any food that you order or eat that doesn't come with fruits or vegetables included. For instance, get fruit (berries, bananas, apples) on your waffles or pancakes. Add green peppers, mushrooms, onions, broccoli, or spinach to your pizza. Put salsa on your salad or sandwich. Slice apples and pears and put grapes in your salads. Put a sliced banana on your peanut butter sandwich. Order a veggie burger instead of a meat burger. Load up any sandwich with cucumbers, tomatoes, lettuce, and sprouts.

3. **Always check the labels when buying food.** See how many calories are in a serving size and also check how many servings are in the entire package that you are considering purchasing. Make sure that the saturated fat and the sugar contents are low. The first listed ingredient on the ingredients label is the one that is the highest concentration in the food that you are buying. If sugars or fats are listed first, then put it back on the shelf.

4. **Restaurant dining.** The increase in obesity seems to coincide with the meals eaten out at restaurants, and not just fast-food restaurants. The portion sizes in restaurants are huge compared to the amount that you eat at home. Skip the French fries, fried foods, cheeseburgers, sodas, and high-fat dressings for salads. Always choose grilled or baked foods without breading. Order hardy vegetable soup whenever possible and avoid cream soups. And, most importantly, don't finish those oversized meals that most restaurants put in front of you. Eat one-half the meal and take the other half home, or share it with a friend.

5. **Eat more frequently.** Small frequent meals keep your body fueled throughout the day and prevent you from overeating at any particular time of day or night. Small meals with lean protein and high fiber added keep your appetite satisfied for hours without any hunger pangs. Adding the lean protein to these small, frequent meals increases your energy level.

6. **Face facts.** To lose weight, you have to eat less. Avoid oversized bowls and plates at home, which tend to hold larger portions. Concentrate on smaller servings and pause during a meal to give your appetite control mechanism time to let you know that you're actually full, and be careful not to eat fast, because you will consume mass quantities of calories before you'll ever know that you're not hungry any longer.

7. **Be careful of soft drinks.** Sweetened soft drinks contain loads of sugar and calories. In addition to sodas, this includes sweetened iced teas, fat-loaded calories in coffee drinks, such as lattes and cappuccinos, and juices that contain little or no juice, but lots of sugar. Stay away from so-called energy drinks, which contain high amounts of sugar and caffeine. These drinks are unhealthy and the energy that they produce initially is from the initial shot of caffeine and glucose absorbed into the bloodstream. These drinks cause unhealthy spikes in both blood sugar and blood insulin, and the high caffeine content of these drinks can be dehydrating. Even diet sodas and teas according to recent studies show that the artificial sweeteners can actually increase your appetite. Switch to fat-free coffee drinks and decaffeinated tea without sugar. Choose 100% low sodium vegetable and tomato juices. Fruit juices are usually high in sugar content even when they sat 100% fruit juice. However, fresh fruits that are combined in a blender are healthy to consume. It's best to also drink lots of water, and occasionally seltzer.

8. **Exercise to burn more calories than you eat.** It's not necessary to join a gym or participate in aerobics classes to burn up fat. You can burn calories by just climbing the stairs, cleaning the house, riding a bike, working in the garden, or just by walking 40 minutes every day. You don't even have to work up a sweat to burn calories while exercising. Studies have proven that people who take a brisk walk for 40 minutes every day burn body fat, improve their physical fitness, and lower their blood pressure, as much as, if not even more than, people who work out at a gym three to four days per week. Even two 20-minute walks per day will give you the same fitness and fat-burning benefits as a 40

minute walk every day. A recent study from a major university showed that sedentary women, in addition to gaining weight their abdomen, buttocks, and thighs, actually increased their deep fat that surrounds the internal organs of the body. This increases the risk of heart disease, hypertension, and diabetes. The study also showed that moderate exercise six times per week for 40 minutes daily, decreased the deep fat by more than 35% and resulted in considerable weight loss over a three-month period.

9. **Drink water** before and during your meal. Water fills you up and decreases your hunger control's appetite center in the brain. You'll naturally eat less food with each meal and feel quite satisfied when you're finished eating. Water is also essential to keeping your metabolism running smoothly and in keeping all of your blood's components in perfect balance. Water also keeps you well hydrated and can prevent spikes in blood insulin levels that cause your blood sugar to drop which subsequently increases your appetite for high sugar bad carbohydrates.

BLAST OFF FAT REALLY FAST!

The typical American diet has a higher fat content than in nearly any other country in the world. There is little doubt that this increased fat intake in our diet is responsible for the development of obesity, as well as many other disorders. It is important to note that fat is the most concentrated source of calories, since a gram of dietary fat supplies your body with **9 calories**. This is compared to only 4 calories contained in each gram of protein or carbohydrate. Since fat has this concentrated source of calories, it is the most fattening type of food that we can consume, and it stands to reason that cutting down on the total fat intake is one of the best ways to cut down on the total amount of calories, and to lose and maintain normal body weight.

Controlling our weight by reducing the amount of saturated fat in our diet has a two-fold benefit. First of all, it will help to control and maintain our weight. Secondly, it will have the beneficial effect of the prevention of cardiovascular and cerebrovascular disease (heart attacks and strokes), since these illnesses have been associated with high levels of blood cholesterol, which, in turn, come from the consumption of saturated fats.

Fat is easily converted into energy. Whereas, almost none of the calories contained in protein in our diets are converted into storage fat cells, almost 95% of the dietary fat can be stored in fat cells when you take in excess calories of fat in your diet. In other words—**it is the fat in your diet that makes you fat.** It is not necessarily the actual number of calories in your diet that makes you fat, it is the number of fat calories that makes you fat. Fat is stored in fat cells called adipose tissue, in a ratio of four parts fat and one part water. Since there are 9 calories in each gram of fat, it means that one pound of fat contains 3,500 calories. It, therefore, takes a deficit, or reduction, of 3,500 calories to lose this one pound of fat.

Fat, unfortunately, can be stored in unlimited quantities. Normal-weight individuals have almost 100,000 calories stored in fat cells. By increasing fat in the diet, combined with a sedentary lifestyle, it is quite easy to add another 50-100,000 calories in fat stores, increasing your weight 15-30 pounds every year. The only way to lose even one pound of body weight is to burn approximately 3,500 calories. This can only be accomplished by cutting back on the total amount of fat in the diet, and also by increasing your physical activity. Nothing else works! Believe me! One of my favorite sayings to my patients when they ask me how to lose weight is: *"The only way you can lose weight is to eat less fat and to walk more, or, if you would like, you can walk more and eat less fat!"*

I am often asked by my patients, "What's the best way to lose weight safely?" There is little doubt that a **low-fat, high-fiber, and lean-protein diet** is the healthiest, safest, and most effective weight reduction program. This plan is designed for quick weight-loss without rebound weight gain. When this diet is combined with walking 40 minutes six days per week and also walking for 40 minutes 3 times per week using hand-held weights (Chapter 10), you have the perfect quick weight-loss & body-shaping plan, where you can blast off fat really fast. *You can actually lose up to 15 pounds and 3 inches in only 21 days on The Philly Fit-Step Walking Diet.*

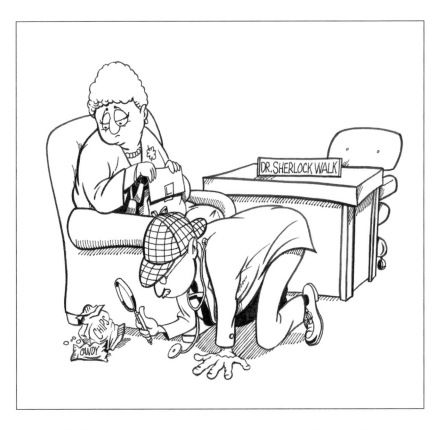

**"My dear Mrs. Hudson, this is certainly not the
healthiest of snacks."**

5

DR. WALK'S WEIGHT-LOSS TIPS

*P*hilly's *Fit-Step® Walking Diet* consists of a series of the Best Weight-Loss & Fitness Tips, which are published regularly in my online publication entitled, *Dr. Walk's Diet & Fitness Newsletter.* I have shared these diet, fitness and health tips with my Philadelphia patients over the past 10 years, many of whom have followed them regularly with excellent weight-loss and fitness results. I have included many of these weight-loss tips in this new book and I hope that you will share the same benefits as my Philadelphia patients have enjoyed over the past decade.

PHILLY'S BEST WEIGHT-LOSS TIPS

WHAT TO THINK ABOUT BEFORE EATING

1. Before food shopping, prepare a list and only go to the market after you've eaten. Going to the market when hungry can lead to impulse purchases of high fat snack foods. Buy only those items on your list. Don't deviate from this list with snack foods, which you might have a tendency to buy, if you had not eaten prior to shopping.

2. When shopping for packaged or canned goods, make sure the item of food you are purchasing has no more than 1.5–2.0 grams of total fat per serving. If it is higher, compare other brands. Always look for non-fat or low-fat products; however, read the fat content on the nutritional label, and don't depend on a label that says "low-fat food." Many so-called low-fat items are fairly high in total fat content; for example 2% milk has 5 grams of fat, and 98% fat free yogurt can have 3.5 to 4 grams of total fat. Always choose foods that are less than 2.0 grams of total fat. Also watch out for labels that say "cholesterol-free." These foods may have 0 grams of cholesterol; however, they may contain many grams of total fat.

3. Foods should be kept out of sight, in your refrigerator or pantry, between meals. Do not place serving dishes on the table during meals to reduce temptation to take second helpings.

4. Don't skip meals. Skipping meals lowers your blood sugar, which brings on cravings for high-carbohydrate, high calorie foods. Eating 3 to 5 small meals per day is far better than eating one or two large meals. When your blood sugar remains constant, you are less likely to overeat.

5. Eat meals more slowly. Take smaller, less frequent bites and chew each mouthful for a longer period of time. Pause between each section of the meal. If you are still hungry when you are finished your first portion, wait at least 15 minutes to see whether or not you really want more. Leave the table as soon as you are finished eating and spend less time in the kitchen or areas that remind you of eating.

6. Restrict your meals to one or two locations in the home for eating to avoid eating in every room. This will reduce the tendency to snack during the day.

7. Individuals who skip breakfast usually wind up with a high fat, high-sugar snack mid-morning: the coffee break with doughnut. A high fiber, low-fat cereal with fruit and skim milk will hold you comfortably until lunchtime.

8. Don't use food as a stress reliever. People have a tendency to seek out high-fat, high-sugar foods when under stress. Substitute music, reading, walking, meditation or a warm bath for food cravings.

9. Don't start a weight reduction program just prior to the holiday season or before vacation time since these are the most unsuccessful times to begin this type of project. The most important part of any successful diet is starting it. Once you've made up your mind to begin your diet, you're half way there. You must be ready from the very beginning to discipline yourself. Just like every other part of your life, discipline is a must!

10. Dining out is difficult whether you are with company or whether you are alone. The reasons are that the portions are at least, two to three times larger in restaurants than they would be at home, and also it seems that most restaurants seem to add high-fat sauces and dressings to everything they serve, in order to make their dishes appear unique. Always request the sauce or dressing on the side and don't be afraid to leave half the dinner on your plate (take it home for another meal.

FOOD SELECTION AND PREPARATION

1. Eat salad greens and vegetables before the main course since these will take the edge off your hunger for higher calorie meat, poultry and fish portions. Substitute non-fat salad dressings or non-fat mayonnaise for regular varieties of these condiments. If not available, either use no dressing, or keep a small portion of dressing on the side and just dip your fork gently into the dressing every 2-3 bites of salad to get the taste without the added fat calories.

2. Soups and stews can be loaded with hidden fats. Refrigerate them overnight after preparing, and skim off the layer of fat that is lying on the surface of the stew or soup. This will remove more than 75% of the fat contained in these products. Choose soups loaded with vegetables and beans, and avoid any soups that are cream-based.

3. Breads that are high in fiber, low in fat are the following: whole grain, bran-enriched, cracked wheat, whole-wheat pita, rye, pumpernickel and those labeled "high fiber breads." Avoid the high fat, low fiber breads: French, Italian, white, garlic bread, rolls and bagels. Remember to check the ingredients label. If the first ingredient doesn't say "whole," then it is not a whole-grain, high fiber bread. Choose whole wheat or oat bran English muffins, whole-wheat rolls or bread, whole wheat or oat bran bagels or raisin bread instead of sweet rolls, doughnuts, cakes and white bread. Remember to always scoop out the inside of rolls or bagels. Use jelly, honey, fruit preserves and all fruit jams, instead of margarine or butter, as spreads for your breads.

4. Make your meals attractive with colorful foods, garnishes and greens, such as carrots, tomatoes, broccoli, spinach, peppers, yams, celery, and parsley, in order to make them more appealing. Also vary your menu plans daily to avoid boredom. Remember that the more colorful the foods are, the more phyto-nutrients they contain.

5. Fresh vegetables and fruits are better choices than canned fruits and vegetables, which can be loaded with salt or sugar. Fruits and vegetable skins are excellent sources of fiber, as are the seeds, (berries, tomatoes, cucumbers, and pumpkins). Steamed vegetables, with or without herbs, can be cooked in a basket over boiling water. Steaming retains the flavor, color and nutrients of the vegetable. Also, foods that require a lot of chewing will leave you with a greater feeling of satisfaction because they take a longer time to swallow and absorb.

6. Fresh or canned beans of any variety are excellent sources of fiber and vitamins. Their low fat content makes them excellent companions to any meal. Make sure they are not prepared with meat (example: baked beans with bacon). Avoid high fat refried beans, but non-fat refried beans are okay.

7. Low fat, non-fat, or part skim-milk cheeses should be substituted for all other cheese. Make sure, however, that you check the total

fat content per serving size. Non-fat yogurt is an excellent source of calcium and its lactobacillus, and other cultures are friendly bacteria for your colon. Cream, whole milk or powdered creamers should be avoided in coffee or tea; substitute skim milk or non-fat dairy creams

8. Peeling a potato (white or sweet) before cooking or eating removes more than 25% of its nutrients and 35-40% of its fiber. A baked potato is an excellent food for meals or snacks (high fiber, low fat), compared to French fries, which are saturated with up to 15 grams of fat per serving. However, if you have a craving for French fries, you can prepare low-fat French fries by thinly slicing potatoes, spraying with non-fat vegetable spray, and baking for 20-30 minutes in an oven at approximately 300 degrees, or microwaving for 3 to 5 minutes. Keep your portion size small.

9. If you put salt on poultry, fish or meat before cooking, the food loses a good portion of its vitamin and mineral content during the cooking process. This is because the added salt causes the food to be drained of its nutrients during the cooking process, which end up in the cooking broth.

10. Trim all visible skin and fat from poultry (white meat), fish and from very lean meats before cooking. Grill or broil poultry, fish and lean meat. Use a light dusting of olive oil or an olive oil spray.

11. Non-stick pans use less fat than cast iron, copper or aluminum pans. Use non-stick vegetable sprays as your first choice; otherwise, a small amount of olive oil (1 tsp.) or canola oil can be used for cooking.

12. Microwaving uses the food's own moisture to cook. It's quick and easy, and you don't have to add any fat when microwaving. Almost all foods are microwaveable.

13. Stir-frying in a pan or wok is a fast way to make tasty vegetables, chicken, meats or fish. Add very small amounts of olive or peanut oil and seasonings followed by either defatted chicken broth or low-sodium soy sauce.

14. Sautéing: Use non-stick, non-fat vegetable sprays or a small amount of wine or defatted broth. Vegetables, fish, poultry or meats are mixed together in a pan. Then add herbs, such as thyme, basil, sage, or dill, for added taste.

15. Avoid sugary sodas, teas, juices and fruit drinks. Avoid drinking a lot of artificially sweetened drinks as they can increase your appetite, due to the hypoglycemic effect (it lowers your blood sugar). Unfortunately for many dieters, new research from Purdue University suggests that artificial or natural sugar substitutes may cause weight gain, because of the spikes in blood insulin levels caused by these non-caloric sugar-free substitutes. Always make plain old water (tap or bottled) your drink of choice.

SNACKS AND DESSERTS

1. A tasty non-fat dessert is **angel food cake** with fresh fruit and non-fat whipped cream. (A slice of cheese or chocolate cake has up to 14 grams of fat). The angel food cake, as described above, has less than 1.5 grams of fat.

2. **Sherbet, sorbet, frozen fruit bars and non-fat frozen yogurts** are excellent substitutes for your ice cream sweet tooth.

3. **Non-fat popcorn** is an excellent low-fat, high fiber snack. Don't add butter or salt. Use hot air popper or microwaveable non-fat varieties. Other low-fat snacks include hard pretzels (non-fat), and flavored rice cakes.

4. Excellent fat-free **fruit and veggie** snack-food choices include dried or fresh fruits, raisins, peaches, apples, plums, apricots, bananas, baby carrots, and celery stalks.

5. **Nuts are packed with nutrition and because of their protein content** are very filling. They contain vitamin E, B-complex, folic acid, fiber, omega-3 fatty acids, and arginine (an amino acid). These nutrients contained in nuts have been shown to reduce bad LDL cholesterol and increase good HDL cholesterol and therefore help to reduce the incidence of heart disease and strokes. The nutrients

in nuts also protect the heart against irregular heart rhythms and help to maintain your blood vessels natural elasticity. A handful of almonds or cashews with a mini-box of raisins make a great tasting healthy snack.

6. **Chocolate**, particularly dark chocolate contains healthful nutrients called *flavonoids*. These flavonoids are antioxidants that protect your heart from dangerous free radicals that can damage heart cells. These flavonoids also protect you from heart disease by decreasing the LDL bad cholesterol and increasing the HDL good cholesterol in the body.

Chocolate also raises blood levels of endorphins (feeling-good hormones), which helps to relax you from anxiety and stress. Dark chocolate also contains traces of a neurotransmitter called anandamide, which produces a feeling of euphoria.

Chocolate also contains health promoting *anti-oxidants* (polyphenols and resveratrol), which can reduce the risk of blood clots that can cause strokes and heart attacks These antioxidants also produce an enzyme called endothelial nitric oxide synthase (ENOS), which relaxes the blood vessels thus lowering your blood pressure. Dark chocolate also contains heart-healthy antioxidants, which have been shown to lower the blood pressure and prevent clots from forming in the brain and heart.

Chocolate is a great appetite suppressant, since it easily satisfies your appetite with just a small amount of its sweet taste. Also, chocolate is actually good for a weight-loss program, because by just eating a small amount of dark chocolate, your appetite-control mechanism is quickly satisfied. Look for dark chocolate with the lowest content of total fat.

7. Low-fat, low sugar, high-fiber **granola bars** with real fruit, are satisfying low calorie, highly nutritious snacks.

8. **A root beer float** is a great satisfying drink to have as a snack. Use diet root beer and non-fat frozen vanilla yogurt in a tall ice cream glass.

9. **Sugar-free Jell-O**, or sugar-free, fat-free pudding, topped with fat-free whipped cream is a tasty, sweet-tooth satisfying snack.

10. A **smoothie** made in the blender with all kinds of fruits, veggies, frozen non-fat yogurt or non-fat milk, and 1 tsp. of wheat germ, and protein whey or soy powder, is a healthy low fat, high protein, appetite satisfying snack.

EATING WHEN AWAY FROM HOME

1. When **eating out**, choose low-fat foods without sauces, like broiled fish or chicken with a large tossed salad. Avoid alcohol, since it can increase your appetite, and add extra calories. Incidentally, one gram of alcohol contains 9 calories, higher than a gram of fat, carbohydrate, or protein. If you like a drink with dinner, a wine spritzer is a good substitute, which is relatively low in total calorie value. Red wine (4 oz.) or a light beer every other night is also acceptable.

2. Don't be afraid to **send back your meal** in a restaurant if they didn't follow your order instructions. If you asked for steamed vegetables, baked potato, and broiled fish without butter, that's the way it should arrive on your plate.

3. At **weddings and other parties** choose the fresh vegetables and fruits without the dips. Avoid those fat-laden little appetizers with toothpicks in them. Consider the toothpicks red warning flags to stay away!

4. When **traveling by air**, order ahead for a low-fat meal when making reservations. They're available! Otherwise, if it is a short flight, have a low-fat snack prior to boarding.

5. **Italian:** Spaghetti or linguini is lower in fat than wider pastas that are often made with eggs. Try to order (when dining out) or buy whole grain pasta or spinach noodles for their high-fiber content. Stick to tomato or marinara sauces (however, some have too much oil, and you can have the waiter drain the oil from the pasta and bring back your dish). Seafood-based sauces without cream are also good substitutes.

6. **Pizza** can be ordered without cheese (tomato pie) and then add on a variety of fresh vegetables. If you want cheese, sprinkle on a little Parmesan cheese. Always blot off the extra fat on top of the pizza with a paper towel or napkin to absorb fat. By using this tip you can remove more than 50% of the additional fat calories from the pizza.

7. **Chinese restaurants:** Stir-fry foods are better than deep-fried. Choose dishes with grains and vegetables. Order brown rice instead of white rice for the extra fiber content (not fried rice, which also comes out brown in color but is low in fiber). Ask to have your food prepared without soy sauce or MSG. Choose vegetable wonton soup or any vegetable-based soup rather than meat-based soups.

8. **Mexican foods** are great, if you can stay away from the deep-fried tortilla chips and order oven-baked chips with salsa instead. Skip the sour cream and guacamole (avocado), both of which are high in fat. Soft corn tortillas (tostadas or enchiladas) with chicken, tomato sauce and onions are good low-fat choices. Burritos or fajitas without sour cream or guacamole are excellent choices with lettuce, tomato and onion, and can be considered low-fat dishes. Avoid regular refried beans, deep-fried chimichangas, beef taco salad and deep-fried tortilla chips.

9. Three-four ounces of **red wine** every other day is heart healthy since the red grapes contain resveratrol, a super antioxidant which helps to prevent strokes, blood clots, hypertension and heart disease, this providing that you have no underlying liver or cardiac problems which prevents consumption of any alcoholic beverages. You can get the same benefits by eating red grapes or purple grape juice without the alcohol.

10. Once again, remember that drinking lots of **water** helps to satisfy your hunger mechanism by filling you up either before or during a meal. The water will help you eat less at each meal, since your stomach will not know whether it's food or water that's in your stomach. Drinking 6-8 ounces of water a day is a great way to

keep your appetite satisfied and help you lose weight. Water is one of the best diet foods, since it contains no calories and satisfies your hunger quickly. Water also fuels your body's energy level, since all of the body's metabolic processes require a constant supply of water to function efficiently.

CALORIES DON'T COUNT—YES THEY DO!

According to a recent study in the *Journal of the American Medical Association,* there is a no magic formula to losing weight. You can lose weight by following a variety of different diet programs; however, the one thing that always counts is the number of calories that you consume vs. the number of calories that you burn daily.

Yes, even those horrendous, low-carbohydrate diets work also, but that's because they restrict calories also, not just carbohydrates. Also, they work because you are creating an unhealthy condition found in diabetics called ketosis, where you are burning protein instead of fat to lose weight. Unfortunately, the weight comes back twice as fast when you stop the diet, if, however, you are fortunate enough not to have damaged your liver or kidneys while you were on this stupid diet.

Unfortunately, Americans have been gaining so much weight in the last twenty years that obesity is becoming an actual epidemic. Over 60% of adults are overweight, which includes approximately 30% who are considered obese. This trend has almost tripled in teenagers during this same time period.

After reviewing over one hundred diet studies since 1999, the researchers concluded that if you want to lose weight, you should consume fewer calories daily over a long period of time. By restricting one type of food over another, as in the low-carbohydrate diets or high-protein diets, you are essentially making a weight loss program more difficult, and essentially more dangerous.

A low-fat, high-fiber diet with moderate amounts of protein and complex carbohydrates is the single, best healthy weight loss diet that you can follow for good health and permanent weight loss. There are no dangerous side effects, no feelings of hunger, and along with permanent weight loss, you have the added benefit of a diet that is actually good for you. You will have less weight, less heart disease and hypertension, less strokes and dementia, and a lower incidence of several forms of cancer. This diet, by its very nature, turns out to be a low-calorie diet in disguise, and what's more, it actually works and keeps on working.

Food Journal

It is important to keep track of when and what you eat at each and every meal, including snacks. It is just as important to be conscious of why you eat, especially when you are nibbling snacks unconsciously throughout the day, or eating more calories than you should consume at meal time. For example, were you watching TV and not paying attention to what you were eating. Were you in a meeting or at work or talking on the phone and eating junk food without really noticing what you were eating?

A food journal can help you solve these problem areas by keeping an accurate record of what you actually eat at each and every meal on each and every day. This record will enable you to establish a more realistic diet plan as you move forward on your Fit-Step Diet weight loss plan.

You can keep your record of your food diary in a notebook or you can do it online at www.myfooddiary.com. To count the total number of calories and the number of grams of fat that you consume at each meal, you can consult any one of a number of food nutrition books, or you can go to any of the websites that list the calories of different foods and also lists the number of grams of carbohydrate, protein, and fat for each food. A food journal gives you a basic guideline of what you have been doing wrong and the means to correct your food eating habits. Make sure that you record everything that you consumed in any given 24 hour period. This record will enable you to establish a more realistic diet plan as you move forward on your Fit-Step Walking Diet.

WOMEN GAIN WEIGHT MORE EASILY THAN MEN

Unfortunately, women gain weight easier and faster than men, which is partially due to a woman's slower metabolism. Men have more muscle mass and burn fat at a faster rate than women. So it is important that women exercise regularly in order to burn calories and to increase their metabolic rates. Women, however, have a distinct advantage over men in that they naturally have more sustained endurance when they exercise. So that women who engage in a regular sustained aerobic exercise program burn more fat calories than men who do strenuous exercises for short periods of time, since quick bursts of energy burn primarily carbohydrates rather than fat. Therefore, sustained aerobic exercise helps women increase their metabolic rates during exercise and also at rest.

It also takes longer for a woman to digest food than it does for a man. Because of the slower production of certain digestive enzymes, women metabolize fat and a number of medications including alcohol at a slower rate than men. Fat in a woman's diet therefore causes her to gain weight easily because of this inability to digest and metabolize fat quickly.

So it's no wonder that fat in a woman's diet is just about the worst thing that she can have in order to lose weight and stay healthy. Fat contains 9 calories per gram, and combined with a women's slower rate of metabolism, considerably more fat is stored in her fat cells.

Increasing lean protein and complex carbohydrates into a woman's diet and reducing saturated fats makes it much easier for her to digest and absorb food for the maximum weight-loss effect.

Low carbohydrate diets, which are essentially high fat diets, make it even more difficult for women to lose weight, and, in particular, to keep the weight off. These diets don't work and they are very toxic to your body. Initial weight loss is always followed by marked rebound weight gain.

FISH: GOOD LOW FAT NUTRITION

Seafood is a good source of high-quality protein, nutrients and omega-3 fatty acids, which is an important part of a well-balanced healthful diet. Omega-3 fatty acids contain DHA and EPA which are the nutrients which give the omega-3 fatty acids their health benefits. Also, fish is a great diet food since it is low in calories and saturated fat, high in protein and contains the heart-protecting, cancer-fighting benefits of omega-3 fatty acids. Even though shellfish has higher levels of cholesterol than other types of fish, it is low in saturated fat and therefore does not raise your blood cholesterol.

The fish oils contained in fish such as wild salmon (better than farm raised), tuna, haddock, sardines, and mackerel contain a lot of **omega-3 fatty acids**, have been recently found to improve exercise induced asthma These omega-3 fatty acids appear to reduce the risk of heart disease, hypertension, strokes, blood clots, degenerative diseases of aging and some forms of cancer. Fatty fish are also low in total saturated fat and calories and satisfies your appetite easily due to its lean protein content. Poaching fish in water at a simmer (just below the boiling point of water) preserves the taste and texture of the fish. Any condiments can be added to the liquid to enhance the flavor, such as garlic or herbs. Fish are low in calories and total saturated fats and are essential for an effective weight reduction program. Eat fish three to four times per week, whether at home or in a restaurant, for a healthy, low-fat, high-protein, great diet tip.

Recent research has shown that these omega-3 fatty acids appear to reduce the risk of coronary heart disease and may help to lower blood fats known as triglycerides. They have also been shown to reduce the risk of high blood pressure, heart arrhythmias, and the formation of blood clots. Omega-3 fatty acids also help to reduce the risk of depression, some neurological diseases of aging such as Alzheimer's disease, asthma, arthritis, and certain forms of cancer (colon, breast, uterus and prostate). *Recent studies show that these health benefits only occur when eating foods that are high in omega-3 fatty acids, and not by taking fish oil supplements.*

Fish is low in calories, low in fat, and high in protein, which makes them ideal for any real weight loss plan. Even shellfish with its higher content of cholesterol is still an important fat-burning food in your diet program. The low saturated fat content of shellfish offsets any cholesterol that these products may contain. The high protein content in fish acts as the fat-burner, since the protein increases your basal metabolic rate. Fat is subsequently burned more quickly and weight loss becomes quick and easy.

PORTION CONTROL TIPS

1. If you find that you have to eat at a fast food restaurant, order a junior or children's hamburger without the cheese. Skip the fries and add a diet soda or unsweetened iced tea to your sandwich.

2. At a restaurant, if you can split a meal with a friend or relative, try to do so, even if there's a sharing charge. Also split a dessert with your companion to enjoy the sweet taste without eating extra calories.

3. If you order in, don't eat out of the container, like when you order Chinese food, or you'll eat the whole portion. Put the different foods on plates, and eat one half the amount of each food and refrigerate the rest for the next day. If you order a pizza, unless there are several people present; take out one or two slices and refrigerate the rest.

4. If you take lunch to work, take a half of a sandwich and a cup of soup to lunch or a big mixed salad without the dressing.

5. If you eat a snack at home, don't eat out of the container that the food came in, like a bag of chips, pretzels, or a container of ice cream or dessert. Serve a small portion in a bowl, and stop before you feel full.

6. Don't be tempted by your dining companions to order similar foods or drinks, especially if they fall outside the parameters of the Diet-Step: 40/40 weight-loss plan.

7. Drink one cup of fat-free milk instead of one cup of whole milk. Add nonfat milk to your coffee, cappuccino, or lattes.

8. Use 1 tablespoon of mustard, ketchup, or fat-free mayonnaise instead of regular mayonnaise in salads or on sandwiches. Mix ketchup and nonfat mayonnaise to make a delicious Russian dressing. Served on a wedge of iceberg lettuce, it makes a tasty snack.

9. Share a small bag of potato chips or French fries with a friend, or skip them altogether, or just taste three or four and throw the bag away.

10. Cut a slice of pizza in half and save the other half for later in the day. Also, blot the pizza with a few napkins to absorb the extra fat and calories

11. Check serving sizes of your favorite foods when you eat out. For example:

    a. One-half cup of cooked cereal or pasta at home is equivalent to a single serving size; however, restaurant portions are equivalent to approximately three serving sizes, and that's before they even add the sauce.

    b. One-half of a bagel is one serving, but a deli bagel is equivalent to at least three servings.

    c. One small pancake or waffle at home is equal to one serving size, but in a restaurant, one pancake is about two and one-half servings.

    d. A dozen potato chips or tortilla chips equal approximately one serving; however, a small bag contains at least two to three servings.

12. Always check the serving sizes on any prepackaged food that you get. You will be surprised that some of them say that the contents contain two or three serving sizes. When most people consume a package of processed foods, they assume that it is one serving size, when, in actuality, it may be two to three serving sizes.

PHILLY'S FAST FOOD TIPS

Most fast foods, especially those found in fast food restaurant chains, are so high in calories, saturated fats, and sodium that they not only contribute to obesity, but they also cause the buildup of fat in your arteries, which may be responsible for the development of heart attacks, strokes, and high blood pressure. These fast food restaurants are a major source of childhood and adolescent obesity not only in Philadelphia, but in the rest of the country as well.

THE WORST FAST FOODS

1. The average double cheeseburger, with large fries and a large soda, contains approximately 1,800-2,000 calories, and approximately 100 grams of fat, of which almost 40 grams are saturated fat. It also contains approximately 1,500 mg of sodium. So, for most people, that amounts to the number of calories that they would consume in one day and three to four times the amount of fat and salt that they would consume in any given day.

2. Two slices of pizza with extra cheese and meat contain 750-800 calories, 35-40 grams of fat (15 grams of saturated fat), and 2,000 mg of sodium.

3. Fried fish sandwiches contain approximately 900 calories, 40 grams of fat (15 grams saturated fat), and 1,200 mg of sodium.

4. Nachos with cheese and sour cream contain 1,200-1,300 calories, 80 grams of fat (25 grams saturated fat), and 2,500 mg of salt.

5. A chocolate milkshake contains almost 800 calories and 40 grams of fat, of which 25 grams are saturated.

6. A large coke contains 200 calories.

7. Large fries contain 600+ calories, 20 grams of fat, and 10-12 grams of saturated fat.

8. Fried chicken or fried chicken wrap with cheese and sauce contains 700 calories and 44 grams of fat (12 grams of saturated fat), and 2,000 mg of salt.

THE BEST FAST FOODS

1. A whole wheat bagel with light cream cheese.

2. Order a grilled chicken sandwich without the mayo or better yet, a grilled chicken Caesar salad with fat-free dressing on the side.

3. A good choice is a small vegetarian chili without cheese.

4. Soft chicken taco without sauce.

5. Order a large salad plain, or add grilled chicken, and add fat-free dressing on the side.

6. Sliced lean roast beef sandwich without the sauce.

7. If you must have fries, order the smallest bag possible without added salt and either split with a friend or toss one-half in the trash before you start to eat.

8. Baked potato chips without hydrogenated oils or trans-fats are low in saturated fats and calories.

9. In spite of #2 on the previous page, pizza can also be a great "fast food." According to *Harvard School of Public Health*, tomato sauce contains an antioxidant called *lycopene*, which has been proven to reduce the risk of heart disease and certain forms of cancer, including breast and prostate cancer. A study of over 5,000 people showed that those who ate pizza one to two times per week decreased their risk of different forms of cancer by over 50%. This antioxidant also is a blood pressure and cholesterol lowering agent. Tomato sauce has more lycopene than just ordinary tomatoes, since it is thought to be the heating process of tomatoes that releases more of the healthy lycopene into the tomato sauce.

Pizza is also more filling than many foods, causing you to eat fewer calories and become appetite-satisfied earlier. You can bump up the lycopene content and decrease the calorie content of pizza by ordering your pizza with light or no cheese, and extra tomato sauce. Or you can order a tomato pie or pizza without cheese. If you do order a regular pizza; make sure you use several napkins to blot up the extra fat before eating. You can reduce the total calorie content of each piece of pizza by more than 25% by using this fat-blotting napkin method. Although pizza, in general, has a lot of calories, there are ways to make it a healthful, low calorie food. Adding lots of veggies to a slice of pizza increases its health benefits, providing you stay away from unhealthy toppings like Pepperoni and sausage. So, all in all, a slice of pizza can be a healthy, low fat food to add to your diet, provided you follow the above guidelines.

10. By far, one of the best fast food snacks in Philly is a soft pretzel known as the SUPERPRETZEL®. It is a great low-fat, low calorie, satisfying snack. These soft pretzels are sold in most foods stores, mini-markets, fast-food restaurants, and sports stadiums. They are also found in the frozen-food section of your supermarket or grocery store. This soft pretzel is very filling, and even if you only eat a portion of it, your hunger mechanism will be promptly satisfied.

The SUPERPRETZEL® found in the frozen food section of the market contains 34 grams of Total Carbohydrate, 1 gram of Dietary Fiber, and 5 grams of Total Protein. They are also extremely low in fat (1 gram of Total Fat; and zero grams of Cholesterol, Saturated fats and Trans Fat). Without added salt; these pretzels contain only 130 mg. of sodium. A favorite way to enjoy your pretzel is with mustard, to enhance its flavor. The SUPERPRETZEL® soft pretzel is an excellent appetite-satisfying, low-fat snack.

PROTEIN POWER

HEALTHY PROTEIN

A lean healthy protein intake appears to have a blood pressure lowering effect, particularly when consuming vegetable protein rather than meat protein. Also the unique combination of protein and calcium in non-fat or low fat dairy products helps to keep your appetite satisfied for a relatively long period of time. Also, this calcium and protein combination found in dairy products appears to increase the metabolic rate and burn fat calories at a faster rate.

It is important to add lean, healthy protein to your diet in the form of fish and poultry without skin, very lean meat; nonfat milk and low fat cheeses, including yogurt; and vegetable protein, including tofu, beans, nuts and legumes. When you are on a low calorie diet, your body needs more protein for the production of energy and your body's cell maintenance. Avoid unhealthy, high fat proteins, such as cheeseburgers, hotdogs, bacon, and butter.

Protein is the essential nutrient responsible for the maintenance and repair of all your organs, tissues, muscles, bones and brain cells. All foods are sources of energy; however, protein provides a greater boost in energy levels since it is absorbed slowly and thus produces a constant source of energy.

HEALTHY PROTEIN MEALS

Balance your meals by adding a small amount of lean protein to each meal:

1. Hard-boiled egg on a slice of whole wheat bread or English muffin.

2. Tuna melt with low fat cheese on whole wheat bread with tomato slice.

3. Small Caesar salad with Romaine lettuce, low fat Parmesan cheese and an ounce of grilled chicken and low-fat Caesar dressing on the side.

4. One slice of whole wheat bread with a poached egg.

5. A cup of cooked oatmeal or high protein cold cereal with cinnamon and ¼ cup of raisins and non-fat milk.

6. A fried egg with nonfat spray and a slice of whole wheat bread.

7. A veggie burger on whole wheat bread or bun with lettuce, tomato, onion and ketchup or a ½ veggie hoagie on scooped-out Italian roll.

8. A soft corn tortilla with fat free refried beans, shredded low fat cheese, lettuce, tomato and salsa.

9. A slice of pizza topped with veggies and a side salad with non fat dressing on side.

10. 2 ounces lean roast beef with horseradish and small baked potato or yam with skin, 1 cup steamed veggies and small whole wheat roll.

11. One cup of whole wheat spaghetti with 12 clams or mussels, garlic, ⅓ cup white wine, ¾ tsp. olive oil, and large tossed salad.

12. One cup of low fat macaroni and cheese with a cup of zucchini, diced tomatoes, onions and garlic, and a small sweet potato and steamed fresh carrots.

13. Nuts, particularly walnuts and almonds, are rich in monounsaturated fats, and cause the brain to release a hormone which actually shuts down the appetite control mechanism in the brain and prevents hunger. Nuts are also packed with protein and help reduce the risk of heart disease. Some nuts (macadamias, chestnuts and Brazil nuts) are too high in calories and fat, have no real heart health benefits, and can even cause sickness due to contaminants.

14. Turkey breast or white meat of chicken breast on whole wheat with lettuce, tomato and non-fat mayonnaise.

15. Any grilled or poached fresh fish is high in protein.

16. Grilled low fat cheese on whole wheat bread with tomato.

17. Egg white omelette with veggies.

18. Eggs also are a good source of healthy protein and are especially rich in heart and brain healthy omega-3 fatty acids. Previously, eggs were thought to be unhealthy because of their high concentration of cholesterol. Recent studies however, have proven otherwise. In an eight year study of more than 125,000 men and women, there appeared to be no link shown between the consumption of eggs and the risks of stroke or coronary heart disease, except among those people with diabetes. It is interesting to note that women who ate more than one egg per day had the lowest risk of coronary heart disease. Eggs contain many healthy ingredients like lutein and xanthein which help to keep your eyes from developing cataracts and macular degeneration. It's still a good idea to limit your intake of eggs to one egg three or four times a week, and substitute egg whites the rest of the week.

HARMFUL PROTEIN

Most low carbohydrate, high protein diets have you eating 3-4 times more protein than the recommended dietary allowance, and in most cases, the high protein you are actually eating is the harmful, high fat kind. These diets tax your kidneys and leach out calcium from your bones, in addition to contributing to elevated blood cholesterol which leads to heart disease and strokes. Minimize all fatty meats (primarily beef, and liver, pork, lamb, ham, sausage, bacon, scrapple, hot dogs, and lunch-meats). Limit fatty fowl like duck, dark meat of chicken and turkey and the skin of chicken and turkey. Also eliminate whole milk and whole milk dairy products, butter, margarine, solid fat spreads, saturated oils, and limit your intake of most polyunsaturated oils.

BEAT FOOD CRAVINGS

Food cravings are a constant battle in the war against overeating. When your under stress or anxious, you have a tendency to crave high calorie foods and sweets. You can overcome food cravings by eating low calorie, crunchy foods such as celery, carrots, apples, rice cakes, popcorn, nuts, seeds and low fat pretzels. The crunch factor helps to reduce stress and anxiety by relaxing your tense neck and facial muscles. Fruits are also a great way to combat sweet food cravings. Also, lean protein and low fat products, high fiber foods produce good-feeling hormones (endorphins and serotonin), which helps to prevent you from giving in to food cravings for sweets and high fat foods.

People who are anxious or stressed out have a tendency to crave sweets and high-calorie foods. Anxiety and stress cause your adrenal glands and pituitary gland to produce certain hormones that stimulate your brain's hunger mechanism to crave refined sugars and carbohydrates (cakes, pies, doughnuts, and candy bars). These quick-fix carbs tend to quell anxiety temporarily by the sudden rise in blood sugar, which causes a feeling of calm. However, a rapid rise in blood sugar causes a rapid spike in insulin which causes a more rapid drop in blood sugar.

You can beat anxiety and stress food cravings by eating low-calorie, crunchy foods, such as apples, celery, carrot sticks, or low-fat pretzels (whole-wheat or sourdough). The crunch factor gives your stress-induced anxiety time to cool down without causing a rapid rise in your blood sugar. The actual process of chewing causes your facial and neck muscles to relax, which, in turn, relieves stress and tension.

If you are depressed or sad, your first inclination is also to head for the sweet bar instead of the salad bar. The quick-fix of sugar raises the blood sugar, which, in turn, spikes the pancreas's insulin production. High levels of insulin in the blood increase the production of serotonin, which improves your emotional mood. You feel more relaxed and mellow, which is actually how antidepressant drugs work, by increasing your brain's serotonin levels. Unfortunately, serotonin levels plummet after insulin levels drop, and the feeling of sadness and depression quickly returns. To combat this feeling, you can boost your serotonin levels for longer periods of time by eating fruits when you are feeling down. Fruits only gradually increase the level of blood sugar because fruit sugar, or fructose, is slowly absorbed. Insulin levels then become graduated, causing a sustained, long-lived blood and brain serotonin levels.

People who eat because they are bored or just plain tired often eat high-calorie, refined sugar carbohydrate snacks, like cakes and candies, which are readily available and easy to buy or consume. A mocha caffeinated latte may taste good, but the caffeine and sugar interfere with the production of endorphins and serotonin. Instead of feeling relaxed and calm, you will feel edgy and wired. Nuts, particularly almonds and walnuts, are great boredom snacks, since they provide omega-3 fatty acids that can relieve the feelings of fatigue and boredom. Combined with raisins, nuts make the ideal feel-good, energy-boosting snack.

People, on the other hand, who are happy or in a good mood often turn to high-fat, high-carbohydrate foods, like pizza or cheese steaks smothered in onions. These foods contain protein and fat, both of which help to produce good-feeling endorphins. On the other hand, they also produce tons of fat and calories, which help to destroy any well-intentioned diet plan. To cause an increase in the production of endorphins, substitute high-fiber, whole-grain cereals and breads for the refined carbs, and substitute lean protein, low-fat cheeses, yogurt, turkey, chicken, and fish for the extra unwanted fat calories. These complex carbohydrates and high-protein foods produce both endorphins and serotonin to keep your mood happy and euphoric. Boost your mood with less fat and less calories. Be happy!

NUTS ARE PACKED WITH NUTRITION

Nuts contain vitamin E, B-complex, folic acid, fiber, omega-3 fatty acids, and arginine (an amino acid). These nutrients contained in nuts have been shown to reduce blood cholesterol, prevent heart disease and stroke and protect the heart against irregular heart rhythms and help to maintain your blood vessels natural elasticity.

The protein content of nuts satisfies your hunger mechanism quickly so that you consume fewer calories. Frequent consumption of nuts (four to five servings per week) has been shown to reduce the risk of coronary heart disease by as much as 50%. Nuts also have been shown to decrease both the total cholesterol by 5-10% and the LDL cholesterol by 15-20%. A study published in *the Journal of Nutrition* indicated that of all edible plants, walnuts have one of the highest concentrations of antioxidants.

In a more recent study reported in the *Journal of Circulation*, from the Hospital Clinic of Barcelona, Spain, Dr. Emilio Ros said that, "This is the first time a whole food, not its isolated components, has shown this beneficial effect on vascular health." He further stated that, "Walnuts differ from all other nuts because of their high content of alpha-linolenic acid (ALA), a plant-based omega-3 fatty acid, which may provide additional heart-protective properties."

Several other beneficial components of walnuts include: L-arginine, which may be cardio protective by dilating the arteries. Walnuts also contain fiber, folic acid, gamma-tocopherol, and other antioxidants, which also help to prevent atherosclerosis (hardening of the arteries). Actually nuts, particularly walnuts and almonds, which are rich in monounsaturated fats, cause the brain to release a hormone called cholecystokinin, which actually shuts down the appetite control mechanism in the brain and prevents hunger.

Two ounces of almonds is enough to release this appetite-suppressing hormone. The monounsaturated fats contained in nuts also have heart-protective properties. These monounsaturated can lower blood cholesterol, particularly the bad LDL cholesterol, and they can also help to reduce blood pressure. Remember that nuts are high in fat; however, they contain the heart-healthy monounsaturated fats which have been shown to have both health benefits and weight reduction properties. Nuts are packed full of nutrition. They contain folic acid, vitamin D, copper, magnesium, fiber, and healthy monounsaturated fats. You just have to be careful to stay under the 35 grams of total fat per day on the Fit-Step Plan.

There are also **omega-3 fatty acids** present in plant foods, such as **walnuts** and in **flaxseed**. These are known as ALA (alpha-linolenic acid). The body, however, must convert ALA into DHA and EPA in order to have the same health benefits as you get when eating fish.

CALCIUM BURNS FAT AND BUILDS BONES

Several new studies have shown that people who regularly drink skim milk and eat yogurt or have one serving of cheese per day lose an average of 1½ pounds per month, with no additional change in their diets. It is believed that calcium decreases the stores of fat in the fat cells by actually burning stored fat. Also, it is thought that the protein content in milk, yogurt and cheese replaces the fat stored in the fat cells by a unique process of providing extra protein to the body's cells. This combination of calcium and protein which is present in milk, yogurt and cheese helps the body to burn fat and store protein.

Another study at the University of Tennessee suggests that calcium found in these foods actually blocks fat storage in the cells that plump up your abdomen, thighs and hips. This calcium also has the added advantage of increasing your good HDL cholesterol and decreasing your bad LDL cholesterol. Non-fat milk and low-fat cheeses and non-fat or low-fat yogurts have the same amount of minerals, vitamins, protein and calcium as whole milk without the added fat content. And, as far as your diet is concerned, fat-free milk contains only 80 calories per glass and is packed with 220 mg. of calcium.

Several recent research studies have confirmed that people, who consume two to three servings of milk, cheese, or yogurt daily, lost considerably more weight than those individuals who just reduced their calorie intake, while consuming very little in the way of dairy products. If you consume low amounts of calcium-rich dairy foods, your body produces a hormone called **calcitrol** which acts by causing the body to push calcium in your blood stream into your fat cells. This storage of calcium in your fat cells causes the body to burn less fat, thus, making more fat available to be deposited in your fat cells,.

High calcium diets have been proven to inhibit the production of this calcium-regulating hormone, so that the amount of calcium and fat stored in the body's cells actually decreases. This actually causes you to store less fat, and ultimately lose more weight. On the other hand, it has been shown that low calcium diets actually increase this calcium-regulating hormone, which causes both calcium and fat to be stored in the body's cells (adipocytes), and ultimately causes weight to be gained.

Fortunately, by increasing the calcium in your diet, you are suppressing the body's production of the Calcitrol. Even more surprisingly, researchers have found that by decreasing the amount of calories that you consume, combined with the high calcium-rich diet, you can actually double the amount of weight that you lose than if by just cutting calories alone. Low-fat dairy products such as milk, yogurt, cheese, tofu and other low-fat dairy products are just as effective as full-fat dairy products in suppressing the production of Calcitrol. In other words, you get the benefits of calcium to burn excessive calories without adding excess fat to your diet. This calcium-regulating hormone works in conjunction with the protein found in dairy products to burn fat more efficiently and more quickly, which is another reason why low or non-far dairy products help you to lose weight.

Vitamin D which is often combined with calcium in milk has also been shown to be helpful in controlling your appetite. Vitamin D whether contained in milk, or in supplement form, or manufactured in your body by exposure to the sun, appears also to reduce the risk of certain forms of cancer, particularly prostate cancer. The active ingredient in vitamin D is Calcitrol, which appears to slow or inhibit the growth of cancer cells. If you are not able to have sun exposure, particularly in the winter then the recommended daily allowance is 200 IU (ages 20-50); 400 IU (ages 51-70); and 600 IU (over the age of 70).

KEEP OFF THE SCALE—REALLY!

Remember, no one loses weight in a straight line. When you are on a diet, you initially lose weight, and then your weight loss levels off. This occurs even though you are eating exactly the same amount as you were when you lost the initial weight. This leveling-off period or *plateau* is the single most hazardous part of any diet program. The reason is that once you've reach the diet plateau, you begin to become discouraged, and you'll say, "I'm still on the same diet, but I haven't lost a pound in over a week." Discouragement leads to frustration, and next you'll say, "The heck with the diet. I may as well enjoy myself and eat some high fat, low carbohydrate foods, since I haven't lost any additional weight over the past week even though I'm still following the diet." At this point, 90 percent of all diets are doomed to failure, since the weight loss pattern now reverses itself and becomes a *weight gain pattern.*

If you can stick out this plateau period, which incidentally is *always temporary*, you'll be surprised to see that the weight loss begins to pick up speed again. It may take a week or two, at the most, but if you are patient, you will again start to lose those unwanted pounds. No one has ever satisfactorily explained this plateau period; however, physiologists believe that it is probably due to *a temporary readjustment of the body's metabolism* in response to the initial weight loss. No matter what the reason is, however, you will always break through the plateau period, providing you don't become discouraged or frustrated. Weight loss will again resume its downward progress toward your ideal weight goal.

This plateau period is one of the main reasons that I insist that my patients do not weigh themselves daily. In fact, *weighing yourself every day is hazardous to your diet.* The reason for this is twofold. First, when you weigh yourself daily and see that you are losing weight, you become happy and elated, and subconsciously you will eat to celebrate. Secondly, if you see that you are not losing weight as fast as you "think" you should, you become depressed and anxious, and sometime during that day you will subconsciously eat because of frustration. So, the rule of thumb is: *The more you weigh yourself, the more you eat!* Believe me, it is true. I've seen my patients go through this frustrating daily weighing process thousands of times. No one on a diet should weigh herself more than once a week, and then you will get a true measure of the effectiveness of your diet. If you must weigh yourself, then mid-week Wednesday is the best day to weigh yourself each week. Monday and Friday are the worst days for weighing in, since they follow and precede the weekend and lead to frustrating eating binges. It took a long time to gain all of that weight; you can't take it off overnight. Be patient!

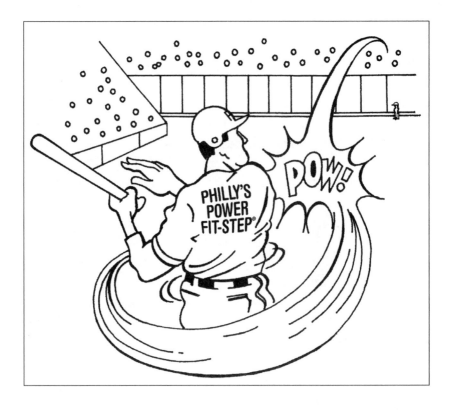

6

POWER FIT-STEP®
IN MINUTES!

T he second component of the Philly Fit-Step Walking Diet is the Fit-Step: 40 minutes six day per week aerobic walking plan. You can divide this walk into two 20 minute sessions if you don't have the time for a 40 minute walk. This part of the Fit-Step Diet Plan is the process that powers up your metabolism to burn calories both during and after you've finished walking. You'll be surprised how good you feel after your 40 minute walk, with increased energy and vigor. The additional flow of oxygen throughout your blood stream will increase your metabolic rate, so that you will burn calories more quickly. This increase in metabolism will allow you to lose weight more quickly and will improve your cardiovascular fitness.

With the advent of the computer age, most people are forced by design to do less and less physical labor. It would seem logical that this would result in more energy being available for other activities. However, how many times have you noticed that the less you do, the more tired you feel, whereas the more active you are, the more energy you have for other activities? Exercise improves the efficiency of the lungs, and the heart and the circulatory system's ability to take in and deliver oxygen throughout the entire body. This oxygen is the catalyst which burns the fuel (food) that we take in to produce energy. Consequently, the more oxygen we take in, the more energy we have for all of our activities.

Oxygen is the vital ingredient, which is necessary for our survival. Since oxygen can't be stored, our cells need a continuous supply in order to remain healthy. Walking increases your body's ability to extract oxygen from the air, so that increased amounts of oxygen are available for every organ, tissue and cell in the body. Walking actually increases the total volume of blood, making more red blood cells available to carry oxygen and nutrition to the tissues, and to remove carbon dioxide and waste products from the body's cells. This increased saturation of the tissues with oxygen is also aided by the opening of small blood vessels, which is another direct result of walking.

So let's take that first power step for energy, fitness and pep. Walking every day will keep a fresh supply of oxygen surging through your blood vessels to all of your body's hungry cells. Don't disappoint these little fellows because you depend on them as much as they depend on you. If you short-change them on their daily oxygen supply, they'll take it out on you in the form of illness and disease. A Fit-Step a day keeps the doctor away.

THE FIT-STEP® POWERS THE DIET-STEP®

Forty minutes walking briskly (approximately 3.5 mph) six days per week, is all that you need to do on the Fit-Step Walking Diet. Or divide your walk into two 20 minute sessions. Either 40 minutes outdoors (walking) or 40 minutes indoors (stationary bike or treadmill) will provide you with maximum cardiovascular fitness, good health, and boundless energy. Remember, this 40 minute walk is a basic part of your weight loss program on the Fit-Step Diet. Your 40 minute walk, 6 days per week is what burns the extra calories needed to lose additional weight and to decrease your appetite when you're on the Fit-Step Diet Plan. If you can't fit 40 minutes into your schedule at one time, then break your walk into two 20 minute sessions throughout the day. The Fit-Step walking plan also provides the fuel that powers your energy level throughout your day. **When you combine the Fit-Step: 40 minute (or two 20 minute sessions) walking plan with the Diet-Step: 40/40 Gm plan, you have the added power to burn additional calories, lose weight, and get fit on the Philly Fit-Step Walking Diet Plan.**

When you first start your Fit-Step walking program, pick a level terrain, since hills place too much strain and stress on your legs, hips and back muscles. Concentrate on maintaining erect posture while walking. Walk with your shoulders relaxed and your arms carried in a relatively low position with natural motion at the elbow. Don't hold your arms too high when you walk, otherwise you will develop muscle spasms and pain in your neck, back and shoulder muscles.

Make sure you walk at a brisk pace (which is approximately 3½ mph) for maximum efficiency. When you begin walking, your respiration and heart rate will automatically become faster; however, if you feel short of breath or tired, then you're probably walking too fast. Remember to stop whenever you are tired or fatigued and then resume walking after resting. Concentrate on walking naturally, putting energy into each step. Soon you will begin to feel relaxed and comfortable as your stride becomes smooth and effortless. Walk with an even steady gait and your own rhythm of walking will automatically develop into an unconscious synchronous movement.

ONLY 21 DAYS TO REACH YOUR PEAK

Your Fit-Step Walking Diet should be planned to meet your individual schedule; however, when you begin it's a good idea to walk at a specific time every day to ensure regularity and consistency. You will be able to vary your schedule once you have started the program. Lunchtime, for example, is an ideal time to plan a 40 minute walk since it combines both calorie burning and calorie reduction. If you have less time for lunch, you'll eat less. If you can't fit 40 minutes into your lunch break, then break up your walk into two 20 minute walks throughout the day.

If you're really out of shape, then you can gradually build up to your 6 day per week, 40 minute walking plan. The 1st week, walk 10 minutes a day, six days per week. The 2nd week, walk 20 minutes a day, six days per week, and the 3rd week walk 30 minutes, 6 days per week. Now you're ready in 21 days for your regular 40 minute walking program, six days per week.

Remember, the speed of walking is not really that important, unless you are walking too slowly (under 2 mph). A brisk walking speed of 3.5 miles per hour is a good walking speed, for maximum calorie burning and aerobic physical fitness. The most important factor is that you walk regularly at a relatively brisk pace. If you become tired easily or get short of breath or develop pain anywhere, or if any other unusual symptoms occur, check with your physician immediately.

THE EXERCISE MYTHS

Why are there so many exercise dropouts? And why don't many men and women even try to begin an exercise plan in the first place? Most people think that an exercise program is futile, since they'll never be able to look like the perfect bodies in the magazines or at the gym. You shouldn't have to feel intimidated by an instructor in a gym or on videotape. Most people think physical fitness is actually harder than it is. And they feel that exercise programs are too complicated, especially when they hear terms like "oxygen consumption," "body fat composition," "body mass index," "lean muscle mass," etc. It actually sounds too complicated and too boring for most men and women to begin exercising in any formalized program.

What most people don't realize is that you don't have to participate in a regimented exercise program to see results. You don't have to join a gym or health club and be intimidated by a twenty-year-old fitness instructor with boundless energy. And you don't have to exercise vigorously or do strenuous exercises in order to obtain maximum fitness and develop a lean, trim body. As we've already discussed, exercise doesn't have to be strenuous to be beneficial. Also, exercise doesn't have to be painful in order to be gainful. Exercise can really be fun! It can be easy to follow and easy to continue. That's why I developed the Philly Fit-Step Walking Diet plan for my Philadelphia patients, so that they could easily become fit and trim, and also easily lose weight. This level of fitness and weight-loss became permanent when they continued the Philly Fit-Step® plan. Now this new program is available for you, and I hope that you'll be as successful as many of my patients have been on the Fit-Step Walking Diet.

No Pain–No Gain Myth

There are two myths about exercising that you should be aware of. The first is the **"No Pain–No Gain"** myth which is completely false. An exercise doesn't have to be painful or strenuous to be beneficial. In fact the reverse is actually true, since it has been shown that moderate exercise is more beneficial than strenuous exercises. Moderate exercises like an aerobic walking program, burn more fat calories than strenuous exercises burn. Strenuous exercises on the other hand, burn more carbohydrates than fats. This fat-burning fact results in a more efficient, long lasting weight-loss with a moderate exercise like walking. Also, there is also the simple fact that moderate exercises do not have the inherent risks of injury that strenuous exercises have associated with them.

Target Heart Rate Zone

The second myth is the **"Target Heart Rate Zone"** myth. No one has ever proved that you have to get your heart rate up to astronomical numbers with strenuous exercises to insure cardiovascular fitness. Moderate exercise actually provides better cardiovascular fitness than strenuous exercise does.

Also, it has been shown that strenuous exercises can do more harm than good when the heart rate is pushed to extremely elevated levels. Cardiac arrhythmias, palpitations, hypertension, and rarely heart attacks and strokes have been reported as being associated with strenuous exercises which stress the cardiovascular system's limits. Walking does not have to increase the heart rate more than 90-110 beats per minutes for maximum cardiovascular fitness.

Both of these so-called exercise precepts are the reason that most people usually want to discontinue their exercise plans or never actually start them in the first place. Once you realize that both of these so-called precepts are in fact myths, and that it is not necessary to engage in painful or stressful exercise, or push your heart beat up to a rapid rate, you can then begin to relax and enjoy the **Philly Fit-Step Walking Diet.**

POWER YOUR ENERGY LEVEL

Once you've reached 40 minutes, six days per week, you will begin to notice the many changes brought about by your improved aerobic fitness and maximum oxygen capacity (the uptake and distribution of oxygen through your body). You will have lots of pep and energy, a trim figure, improved breathing capacity and muscle tone, improved exercise tolerance, a better night's sleep, a feeling of peace and relaxation, and a lessening of tension. Once you start the Philly Fit-Step Walking Diet plan, you will have taken the first steps towards weight-loss, improved cardiovascular fitness, good health and a long, happy life. The great part about walking as an exercise is that you aren't limited to a particular time or location. Walking doesn't require special clothes or equipment. You can walk before or after work, or if you drive to work, you can park your car a block or two from the office, and walk the rest of the way. If you take the bus or train, get off a stop before your station and walk. An enclosed mall could be the perfect place for your walk in bad weather. Remember to take 40 minutes from your lunch break and walk. Just think of how good that fresh air will feel and smell. If you only have 20 minutes, then add on the additional 20 minutes later in the day or early evening. You actually get the same fitness benefits whether you walk for 40 minutes at one time or for 20 minutes twice in the same day.

Each city usually has a guidebook containing historical sites, restaurants, shops of interest; cultural centers and interesting walking tours. There are many excellent books about walking tours and walking paths in Philadelphia which we'll mention shortly. Every city or town has its own books or pamphlets about good walking paths and walking tours, which can be found at your local bookstore. If you live near a park, the country or the seashore, a walking trip will be a refreshing change. Take the time to walk everywhere. Each new area has its own natural beauty. The wonderful world of walking is literally at your feet. Just take that next step for vigor, vim and pep.

INDOOR PHILLY FIT-STEP PLAN

It's not necessary to wait until the "weather is better" to go out and walk. There's no excuse for not exercising at home on any day when the weather is inclement. Also take precautions against exercising when it's very hot or humid outdoors. Heat exhaustion and occasionally heat stroke are complications frequently found in those fanatical runners that you see running on hot, humid days. Remember, it's not necessary to walk outdoors if the weather is extremely cold, windy, wet, hot or humid. Here are various indoor exercise alternatives to help you stay on your Fit-Step Plan

1. STATIONARY FIT-STEP®:

This is a combination of walking and running in place. Walk in place for 5 minutes lifting your foot approximately 4 inches off the floor and taking approximately 60 steps a minute (count only when right foot hits floor). Alternate this with 5 minutes of running in place lifting your foot approximately 8 inches off the floor and taking approximately 90 steps a minute (again only count when the right foot hits the floor). Use a padded exercise mat or a thick rug. Wear a padded sneaker or walking shoe. Bare feet will cause foot and leg injuries. Repeat this walk-run cycle twice daily, for a total of 40 minutes. You can break this up into two 20 minute sessions or four 10 minute sessions. If you tire easily, stop and rest. This is really a boring exercise for most people and the following indoor exercises are much more fun.

2. DANCE FIT-STEP:

Turn on the music and dance to your favorite music, whether it's pop, jazz, classical, R&B, country or any music with a moderately fast beat. Make up your own moves and dance to the beat of the music.

MUSIC BURNS STRESS AND CALORIES

Music can release stress and tension and alleviate anxiety by focusing your thoughts on the music rather than on your problems. Walking to music actually helps you to burn more calories and lose more weight while relieving stress and tension. You can create your own mix of songs to include a warm-up phase, some fast paced tunes, and then mellow music for your cool down phase. Music in the range of 115 to 120 beats per minute is ideal for walking. Let your body naturally adjust to the beat of the individual songs that you are listening to.

You can also work out at home to music while on your stationary bike or treadmill. The faster the music, the faster your workout and the more calories you will burn. If you are not into indoor exercise machines then try dancing to the music at home. Dancing is a whole body exercise that can be as gentle or as vigorous as you like. Any type of dance step will do. It is your preference whether it is tap, jazz, folk, modern or aerobic dance. You can usually find a video which helps you to dance to your favorite type of dance step.

In a study at Farley Dickinson University it was shown that women who exercise to music, in addition to lowering their calorie intake, they lost twice the amount of fat and pounds compared to a group of women who did not listen to music when they exercised. It was thought that those women, who listened to music while exercising, were more motivated and pushed themselves harder during their exercise program than those women who did not listen to music while exercising.

Another recent study showed that people in their 50s and 60s had improved physical fitness, better balance and better flexibility when they danced regularly. You can dance at home, getting lessons from a DVD or online at such sites as learntodance.com, dancetv.com, learning2dance.com, and youtube.com. Or, if you'd like, you can take a class or two at your local gym or Y or at a dance studio in your area. Dancing at home is lots of fun, and a great way to get your 40 minutes of aerobic calorie burning exercise every day.

3. UPRIGHT STATIONARY BIKE:

One of the easiest ways to continue your indoor Fit-Step® program is by using an upright stationary exercise bicycle, in order to travel the indoor road towards fitness and good health. The most important features in a stationary bicycle are a comfortable seat with good support, adjustable handlebars, a chain guard, a quiet pedal and chain, and a solid front wheel. Most come with speedometers to tell the rate that you are pedaling and odometers to tell the mileage that you pedal. An inexpensive stationary bike works just as well as an expensive one. Stationary bikes with moving handlebars are worthless. They claim to exercise the upper half of your body. In reality, they move your arms and back muscles passively, which can result in pulled muscles and strained ligaments.

The stationary bike is one of the safest and most efficient types of indoor exercise equipment that can be used in place of your outdoor walking program. You can listen to music, watch TV, talk on the telephone, or even read (a bookstand attachment can easily be clamped onto the handle bars) while riding your stationary bike. If the bike comes with a tension dial, leave it on zero or minimal tension. Remember, it is not necessary to strain yourself to develop aerobic fitness. Exercises like walking and the stationary bike can be fun, without being painful or stressful. You may alternate days of outdoor walking and indoor cycling depending on your individual schedule.

You should pedal at a comfortable rate of between 10-15 miles/hour. To complete your daily exercise requirements, pedal for 40 minutes every day, which can be divided into two 20 minute sessions to avoid fatigue. Always wear a walking shoe or sneaker (never pedal bare-foot). A chain guard prevents clothing from getting caught in the bike chain; otherwise roll up your sweats.

4. RECUMBENT STATIONARY BIKES:

Some people feel that their body alignment is more comfortable and natural on a recumbent stationary bike. They also tend to say that the bike seats are more comfortable and ergonomically shaped than seats for upright bikes. Some studies have also shown that the recumbent stationary bike puts less stress on the upper and lower back muscles while pedaling. Recumbent bikes also help to build up the quadriceps muscles more than stationary upright bikes because of the positioning of your legs, and are therefore good for individuals with most types of knee problems. It's an individual choice as to which type of bike feels more comfortable for you. Both bikes provide the same level of aerobic fitness and calorie burning.

5. TREADMILLS:

The treadmill is an effective way to burn calories and build cardiovascular fitness. Manual treadmills are hard on the feet, since you have to push down to make them move and the walking motion is unnatural. Look for motorized treadmills with a deck area (the walking space) with enough length and width to accommodate any stride. The deck area should be at least 18 inches wide by 55 inches long. A cushioned deck is better for your ankles and knees and a thick tread belt is best. You can compare the thickness by the feel when you try out the treadmill or by asking the salesman for the thickness measurement, which can then be compared to other treadmills belt's thickness.

Look for motorized treadmills with a high continuous duty rating of at least 1.5 horsepower as opposed to a motor with a maximum output. Continuous duty motors provide you with a constant maximum power, whereas maximum output motors surge to accommodate short spurts, but you won't be able to walk smoothly for an extended period of time. You can also choose a treadmill with a power incline; however, too much of an incline is bad for the knees and ankles and can put a strain on your back. Also, make sure that the machine has an automatic stop button, since, if you stumble or feel dizzy, you can push the button and halt the machine instantly. Exercise for 40 minutes a day either at one time, or divided into two 20 minute sessions. Some people however, find that the treadmill is too hard on their ankles, and especially the knees, because of the constant pounding and impact that the legs endure while on the treadmill. An elliptical machine may be a better choice for these individuals. It should be noted again, that two 20 minute sessions are just as effective as one 40 minute session.

6. WALKING-WHILE-WORKING EXERCISE

Many women and men spend much of the day in front of their computers. It's often difficult to find time during the day to go to a gym, and many people are too tired after a long day at the office to exercise, even at home. There is a unique alternative which will allow you to walk while you are working. It has been shown that you can set up a slow moving treadmill in front of your workstation. Your workstation should be mounted above your treadmill by creating a shelf for your laptop. This type of indoor exercise may be too complicate for most people; however, many business people who don't have the time to exercise during the day have utilized this combo of work and exercise.

You have to go slow on the treadmill at first (approximately 0.5 miles per hour) so that you can type or read without bopping up and down. Set your laptop on the shelf so that your eyes are level with the middle of the screen and your forearms are parallel to the floor. This procedure may take a lot of practice before you can get used to it; however, once mastered, you can burn a lot of calories during the day without sitting at your desk workstation.

To get started, start the process while watching TV first, and then graduate to surfing the Internet, so that you can feel comfortable with your computer. Then gradually start to type, send and receive emails. Follow that process while actually doing your regular work on your computer while walking on the treadmill. For additional tips on this unique form of workout, check out websites such as: www.walking-whileworking.com. You don't need an expensive treadmill for this activity, since you won't be using it for running.

This type of walking while working exercise can also be accomplished more easily using an upright stationary bike, where you hook up your laptop computer to the front of the bike on a stand. Many stationary bikes come with built in stands for books, which can be widened to accommodate a computer. Also remember an additional benefit of walking or riding while working. Work related telephone calls can easily be accomplished while you're exercising. In fact, the added endorphins produced while exercising will give you the added benefit of clear and insightful thinking during your business calls. Many great ideas and plans have been generated by the person who walks or rides while working.

7. ELLIPTICAL FITNESS MACHINES:

This type of machine combines the movement of a treadmill and a stair climber. Your feet loop forward to simulate walking, but the footpads rise and fall with your feet. The elliptical motion provides a no-impact type of exercise, which is great if you have any type of knee or back problem, which makes walking difficult. For maximum exercise, an elliptical machine with dual cross-trainer arms, which you move back and forth as you stride, rather than the stationary arms, provides maximum exercise and burns more calories and uses more muscle groups. Most of these machines come with an adjustable ramp incline and resistance settings. However, the normal setting is usually more than adequate for cardiovascular fitness. Also, be careful of small space-saving elliptical machines, since they may not comfortably accommodate a tall person's stride, or may not afford full range of motion. Try out different machines to see which one you're comfortable with. The elliptical machine can be a very good alternative to outdoor walking. It's best to divide this exercise into two 20 minute sessions, totaling 40 minutes. Some people however, have difficulty getting used to the elliptical machine and feel that the effort required for this type of motion is too strenuous. Try one first to see if they are comfortable to use.

8. SWIMMING:

40 minutes of swimming provides the same aerobic conditioning and cardiovascular fitness benefits as walking and other indoor Fit-Step exercises. Swimming, in fact, has the added benefit of being easy on the joints, especially if you have any form of arthritis or back problems. The reason for this is that swimming puts very little stress on the joints because of the decreased gravity factor provided by the buoyancy of the water. If you have access to an indoor or outdoor swimming pool, then 40 minutes of swimming will fit the bill perfectly for the Fit-Step plan. Remember, you can divide your swim into two 20 minute sessions. Water aerobics are also excellent non-weight-bearing exercises for fitness, weight-loss, and body shaping and helping to prevent osteoporosis.

9. SKIPPING FIT-STEP:

If you're coordinated enough to use a jump rope, skipping can be a fun indoor exercise. Skip over the rope alternating one foot at a time for 5 minutes and then skip using both feet together for 10 minutes. Use a mat or padded rug with a padded low sneaker or walking shoe. You can do this exercise two or three times daily for a total of 40 minutes. Or you can divide this exercise into two 20 minute sessions. If you feel you are not coordinated enough for rope skipping, then skip it!

10. MALL WALKING:

For those of you who don't like to exercise at home when the weather's bad, an indoor mall can be just the place to take your 40 minute walk. Many malls open early before the stores open to accommodate "mall walkers." If you have access to one of these enclosed malls and don't like to stay at home exercising, then by all means, get out there and do the Fit-Step. Remember to put vigor, vim and pep into your mall walk step. Keep your eyes straight ahead so that you won't be window-shopping walking. If you tire easily, then divide your walk into two 20 minute sessions.

TRAVEL FIT WITH THE PHILLY FIT-STEP

Whether you're taking a vacation or a business trip, you can still keep trim and fit with your walking program. Cruise ships and trains are ideal for short walks. Walk around the airport concourse while waiting for flights or during layovers. If you have a long flight, make sure that you get up frequently and walk around the plane. If you're in your seat for any length of time, then move your legs up and down frequently to prevent blood clots from forming. Most major airlines, cruise ships and trains offer special diet menus. If you have to splurge on one meal a day, don't worry. You'll walk it off in no time at all

Most major hotels can give you a map of the area for a walking tour. Get up early before your meeting and take a brisk 40 minute walk. Use the stairs whenever possible and walk around the hotel as much as possible if the weather is bad. Many hotels have small gyms where you can swim or use a stationary bike—take advantage of them if the weather's bad instead of watching TV. Many business trips are associated with a lot of stress and walking can ease away the tension, leaving you more relaxed and more efficient. Speakers always do better after they've had a walk, since they have more brain oxygen and relaxing brain chemicals (endorphins) and less carbon dioxide. This aerobic walk allows you to give a sharp, clear, concise presentation with no stage jitters.

You can keep fit and have lots of pep when you do the Fit-Step.

Don't let a little trip, trip you up. Most people feel exhausted after a vacation or a business trip because they sit around all day and stuff their faces with food and drink. Make it a habit to walk at least 40 minutes every day while you're away. You'll return from your travels feeling fit and rested. And hopefully, you'll weight the same as when you left.

PHILLY'S FIT-STEP TIPS

1. Our bodies are one of the few machines that break down when not in use. A physically active person is one who is both physically and mentally alert. A walking program can actually slow down the aging process and add years to our lives. Walking has been proven to be a significant factor in the prevention of heart and vascular disease. It strengthens the heart muscle, improves the lung's efficiency, and lowers the blood pressure by keeping the blood vessels flexible. Walking will add years to your life, and life to your years! Be sure to get a complete physical exam from your physician before starting any exercise program.

2. In order to walk comfortably and efficiently without tiring, you should balance your body weight over the feet or just slightly ahead of them. Keep your body relaxed, and your knees bent slightly, utilizing a steady, even pace, and a brisk walking stride. To obtain the most benefit out of your walking program you should try to walk with the Fit-Step heel and toe method, pointing your feet straight ahead. The leading leg is brought forward in front of the body, thus enabling the heel of the lead foot to touch the ground just before the ball of the foot and the toes. Your weight is then shifted forward so that when your heel is raised, your toes will push off for the next step. Your arms and shoulders should be relaxed, and they will swing automatically with each stride you take. Before long, you will develop a natural rhythm, pace, and stride as you walk. This Fit-Step® heel and toe walking method uses the calf muscles to pump the blood up the leg veins back to the heart and lungs, and then out through the arteries to all your body's cells, tissues, and organs.

3. When you walk, don't slouch. Walk tall! Walk with your head up, shoulders back, stomach in, and your chest out. Learning to walk tall comes with practice, but after a while, this stance will become a natural part of your walking style. Your stride is the single most important aspect of your walk. There is no correct stride length. Stretch as much as you can without straining when you are walking. Thrust your legs forward briskly, swing your arms vigorously and feel your energy surge forth as you walk with the Fit-Step stride.

4. Keep your pace steady, never push and don't try to accelerate your speed when walking. If you do get tired after a short period of time, stop and rest and then re-start again at a steady and even pace. Don't rush; just walk at a comfortable pace. Your rhythm of walking is a condition that will come naturally as you continue your walking program. Keep your body relaxed and your stride steady and even, and your rhythm will develop naturally. Uneven walking surfaces that you encounter will control your rhythm, especially going down or uphill. Don't fight it, just walk naturally and you'll be doing the Philly Fit-Step.

5. Remember, it's the amount of TIME that you walk every day that is more important than the distance or even the speed. If you walk 40 minutes every day, it doesn't make any difference whether you are walking 2½, 3, 3½ or 4 miles per hour. You are still burning calories, losing weight, and developing physical fitness. In other words, it doesn't matter how far you walk or how fast you walk, as long as you walk regularly. You'll be walking for 40 minutes, 6 days each week to keep your fitness and energy level at its peak. You'll however develop your best fitness level, if you can walk at a brisk pace, which is approximately 3½ miles per hour.

6. Be alert. Be aware of your surroundings. Avoid an area that is un-populated: deserted parks, trails, streets, parking lots, open fields. Vary your route and time of day that you walk. Stick to daylight hours. Walk in familiar or well-populated areas. Plan your route beforehand. If you feel uncomfortable in any area, turn back;

follow your intuition. Let someone know where and when you walk. Carry a cell phone with you at all times. If you're lost, call a friend or the police. If you become tired, stop and rest in a populated area (example: restaurant or a store).

7. If possible, walk with a dog, a friend, or carry a stick, a walking cane, an umbrella, or just a branch for protection. Ignore strangers who ask you questions or call after you. Many stores now also carry walking sticks for dress or protection when you walk. These sticks can also help you climb hills if you are hiking and can act as a handy weapon if you have need to use one.

8. Be careful when you wear MP3, CD, smart phones, or iPod earphones when walking, since they may prevent you from hearing traffic or people coming up behind you. You can also place the ear phones on the bony part of the skull (mastoid bone) directly behind each ear and you'll hear almost as well as if the ear phones covered your ears. Otherwise keep the volume low to be aware of your surroundings. Never trust a moving vehicle! They'll never give you the right-of-way, especially Philadelphia drivers. Don't argue with a car. You'll be the loser.

9. Stay away from areas where people may hide: bushes, parked cars or trucks, alleyways, parking lots, etc. If you are threatened or are suspicious of anyone, run into a shopping center, apartment house, crowded street or just knock on someone's door. Avoid overgrown or wooded areas and dark streets. Stay away from parked vehicles containing strangers. Wear a whistle on a chain or carry a pocket noise alarm. Don't hesitate to use them even if you just suspect trouble.

10. Wear light-colored clothing, especially if walking at dawn or dusk so that you are easily seen by traffic. When clothing is wet it appears darker than when it's dry, so be careful in rainy weather. Wearing reflective material on clothing and shoes while walking after dark or at dusk can mean the difference between a safe walk or a trip to the hospital. Reflective material will increase visibility as much as 200 to 750 feet.

11. Keep a record of your walking program. For example, how long did you walk today, and approximately how far did you walk? Record the time and location of your walk and your impressions of the area in which you walked. Maybe it's an area you'd like to stay away from or one you'd like to explore again. You can wear a pedometer which keeps track of the miles that you walk. They have computerized pedometers that measure steps taken, distance traveled, calories burned, pace, heart rate and timed events. However, an inexpensive non-computerized pedometer works just as well and costs considerably less than the high-tech models.

12. Don't expect results too soon. Whether it's fitness or weight-control that you're looking for, remember, "Rome wasn't built in a day and neither were you." Give your body time to adapt to your regular walking program. Vary your walking program. Vary your walking times (morning, afternoon or evening) depending on your schedule. Make your walking program convenient and flexible. The more adaptable you are to when and where you walk, the more likely you are to do it on a regular basis.

13. Try to walk with a friend or relative for safety. Walking can be a social activity as well as an exercise. Spending time with someone you like or love can certainly add to the enjoyment of your walking program. Walking is one of the only exercises that allows you to talk as you walk. If you are unable to talk because of shortness of breath then you're probably walking too fast. Change your walking route every week or two. Remember to observe any new sights and sounds along your walking path. The road less traveled may be the most fun.

14. Take a 40 minute walk-break instead of a coffee-break or two 20 minute walks instead of two coffee breaks. Walking actually clears the mind and puts vitality and energy back into your body's walking machine. Coffee and a donut add caffeine and sugar to your body's sitting machine. Both the caffeine and sugar cause your insulin production to be increased, and following an initial

rise in blood sugar, there is a sharp drop in your blood sugar from this excess insulin. So instead of coming back to work invigorated as you do from a walk break, you come back fatigued, light-headed and dizzy from a coffee and donut-break.

15. Don't be afraid to take a break for a few days or even a week. Any exercise program, even one that's as easy and fun-filled as walking can eventually become a little tiring. A few days' break from your schedule will give you a short breather so that you can return to your walking program with renewed interest and enthusiasm. Remember, you won't gain all of your weight back or get out of shape if you take an occasional break from your walking program. Never exercise if you are injured or ill. Your body needs time to heal and recuperate from whatever ails you. Remember, you can't exercise through an injury or an illness. Many so-called fitness enthusiasts have tried this with disastrous results. For example, a strained muscle has been aggravated into a fractured bone or a simple cold has turned into pneumonia. Listen to your body.

The Fit-Step walking method is the ideal weight control and fitness program. Studies in human physiology have proven that walking acts as a weight reduction plan without actually dieting and a fitness program without strenuous exercises. Too often today we allow a sedentary lifestyle to dominate our daily living. We sit at our desks all day and in front of the TV set in the evenings. We drive to our destination, no matter how close or how far, instead of doing what's easy, natural and healthful—walking. Most of us would rather spend 20 minutes in our cars waiting at the drive-in window of a bank, rather than getting out and walking the length of the parking lot. Even at work, we opt for the elevator even if it's only for a few floors. At the supermarket or shopping mall most of us would rather drive around the parking lot several times, so that we can get a parking spot closer to the store. These are all good opportunities to do the Fit-Step, not the car-step. Use your feet, not your wheels, and you'll look great and feel full of pep when you do the Fit-Step.

THE HILLS ARE ALIVE WITH THE SOUND OF FITNESS

To burn calories at a faster rate, try walking up an incline, such as a moderate grade hill for a short period of time, say five or ten minutes. Walking up the hill will increase your metabolic rate and you will burn calories at a faster rate then by just walking on a flat surface. You will notice a faster heart rate and faster breathing as you walk up any the incline.

However, you must be in relatively good shape to walk up hills. This means that you should have been on your 40 minute daily walking program for at least six to eight weeks before you attempt to walk up hills. If you become tired or short of breath then stop and rest. You should be able to walk up slightly graded inclines without any discomfort if you are in reasonably good shape. If, however, you find that walking up hills seem too difficult or tires you too easily, then continue your regular walking program on flat surfaces.

Steep hills should definitely be avoided because the risks of ligament and tendon injuries are much more frequent when walking up steep inclines. In particular, it is the down hill descent that makes you more prone to ankle and knee injuries because on the descent your stride is uneven and you start to descend faster because of gravity so that you have to actually drag your heels into the dirt in order to prevent you from accelerating too fast. If your goal is to burn calories at a faster rate and you feel relatively comfortable walking up mild to moderately graded hills, you can make hill climbing a part of your weekly walking program, say for five or ten minutes on two or three days per week.

Remember too that walking up uneven, slightly graded hills can cause leg muscle fatigue and muscle cramps, so be sure to stop walking if your legs cramp up and switch to walking on a flat surface. Hills are only necessary if you feel that you have to speed up your metabolism to burn more calories. Otherwise, you can get the same fat burning boost by just walking on flat surfaces for a longer period of time without the hazards and/or dangers of climbing hills.

I'M GIVING UP! EXERCISE IS BORING

How many times have you heard someone or even perhaps yourself say, **"I'm giving up, exercise is boring!"** Over 65% of women and men who start an exercise program abandon it after 4-6 weeks. Surprising, isn't it? Not really! Initial enthusiasm is often quickly replaced by boredom. Most exercise equipment and athletic clothes quickly find their way into the recesses of the closet. Walking, fortunately, is one of the only exercises that the majority of people stay with. The percentage of men and women who give up walking as a regular form of exercise is less than 25% compared with other forms of exercise programs. Perhaps it's because walking doesn't require special equipment or clothing. Or perhaps it's because there are no clubs to join or dues to pay. Or perhaps it's just that most walkers are usually rugged individualists and are more determined than most people to keep in good shape.

I think the real reason that walkers stay with their walking program is simply that walking is fun! And isn't that what an exercise should be? True, we all want physical fitness, good health, weight control and longevity. But we also want an escape from the stress of everyday living, and that's simply having fun. Walking provides a stress-free, fun-filled activity that we can do anyplace, anywhere, and anytime.

STAY MOTIVATED

Most people, who are overweight or not physically fit, are usually too embarrassed to join a gym. Joining a gym should be the last thing on your mind. All you have to do is take a brisk walk for 40 minutes six days per week, and you're on your way to losing weight and becoming physically fit. If you can't fit 40 minutes at one time into your daily schedule, then try to divide it into two 20 minute sessions a day. Your weight-loss and fitness benefits will be exactly the same as one 40 minute daily walk.

Staying motivated is the key to any successful weight-loss and fitness program. Walking with a companion is one way to stay motivated. Also, by varying the route and location of your walk every couple of days you'll enjoy a fresh perspective on your daily walking exercise. You'll be exposed to new sights, sounds and smells, such as a park with pretty, fragrant flowers and beautiful trees. Also, you'll see different sections of the city or suburbs that you live or work in with a variety of new faces and places.

Another sure-fire way to stay motivated when you walk is to vary the speed or intensity of walking during your walking exercise workout. For instance, speed up your walking pace for 30-60 seconds every 5 to 10 minutes during your 40 minute walk. You'll feel the extra energy pour into your body as you take in additional oxygen with your increased speed of walking. You'll also burn more calories as you speed up your walk, thus increasing your rate of weight-loss and physical fitness. Also, if you walk an extra 5 or 10 minutes a day, you will vary your daily exercise routine as you burn more calories for additional weight-loss and fitness. See Chapter 7 for Quick Weight Loss Walking.

You'll be able to stay motivated when you add the Easy Strength-Training Exercises (Chapter 10), while you're walking for 40 minutes, or two 20 minute sessions, with hand-held weight three times per week. These strength-training exercises help to build upper body muscles as you burn extra calories. By using different upper body muscles while walking with light-weight, hand-held weights, you'll feel the boost of energy surge throughout your body as your metabolic rate increases with this additional muscle activity. You in fact will have a *double blast of calorie burning* with the Philly Fit-Step Diet, while walking with weights. First you'll burn calories by the aerobic activity of walking and secondly you'll burn additional calories by building muscle tissue which actively burns calories. This double blast of calorie burning promotes maximum weight-loss, physical fitness and body shaping.

It's easy to stay motivated with the Philly Fit-Step Walking Diet, since you will find new and exciting places to walk every day, no matter what city or town that you live in. Philadelphia has a number of walking paths in center city's historical areas as well as many of the lovely parks and walking paths dotted throughout the city. There are several excellent books on great walking paths and walking tours in Philadelphia as well as in your own city or town. Philadelphia is one of the most walkable major cities in the United States. Check the Appendix for Famous Landmarks and Walking Tours of Philadelphia.

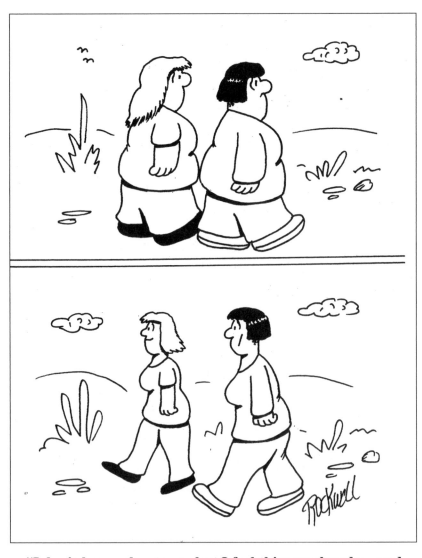

"I don't know about you, but I feel thinner already—and we've only been walking for 40 minutes."

7

DIETWALK®: QUICK WEIGHT-LOSS

THE FAT FORMULA

The latest report from the National Institute of Health again confirmed that obesity is a major health risk. The evidence is strong that obesity not only shortens life, but actually affects the quality of life also. Almost 20 percent of Americans are overweight. How can you tell if you're one of them? It's simple—just follow the **fat formula** for your normal weight:

Females—100 lbs. for the first 5 feet in height, plus 5 lbs. for each additional inch. Example: 5'2" = 110 lbs.

Males—106 lbs. for the first 5 feet in height, plus 6 lbs. for each additional inch. Example: 5' 9" = 160 lbs.

BMI

Body mass index (BMI) is a new measurement of your weight related to your height. It is another way to assess body fat in relation to your height. The BMI is a complicated mathematical formula based on your weight in pounds and your height in inches. It's much easier to consult BMI tables on the internet or in health magazines, than it is to try to figure out this mathematical formula yourself. Generally the BMI also rates your risk of heart disease depending on your body mass index. The following is a general chart **(Table I),** which indicates if you're overweight and your potential risk of heart disease.

TABLE I

BMI	WEIGHT	HEART DISEASE RISK
18.5-24.9	Normal	None
25.0-29.9	Overweight	Increased
30.0-34.0	Minimal Obesity	High
35.0-39.9	Moderate Obesity	Very High
40.0 or greater	Extremely Obese	Extremely High

If you flunk the fat formula or the BMI, then you really need to start to walking-off weight using the **DIETWALK QUICK WEIGHT-LOSS WALKING PLANS.** The increased medical risks for being overweight are: hypertension, heart attacks, strokes, diabetes, arthritis, cancer of all types, and increased surgical risks if you happen to need an operation. These risks seem to be even worse if most of your weight is carried in the upper body (chest, hips and abdomen) rather than in the buttocks and legs.

DIETS DON'T REALLY WORK

Consumer Reports polled 95,000 subscribers who tried to lose weight over the last three to five years. Over 19,000 subscribers used commercially supervised diet programs, and the rest tried to lose weight on their own. The results of both groups were similar, in that dieters lost an average of 10-12 pounds while on their respective diets. The discouraging news, however, is that most of the respondents to this survey regained almost one-half of their weight loss in the first three to six months after ending the diet program, and two-thirds of the weight was regained in two years. Only 20% of these dieters were able to keep off two-thirds of the weight they had lost for more than a two-year period. Many of these commercial diet programs cost an average of $65-70 per week—a pretty hefty price to pay for a temporary weight loss plan.

Most women are more likely to perceive themselves as fat, whereas in reality, men are more likely to be overweight. In a recent Harris poll of over 1,200 women and men nationwide, the findings were as follows:

- Over 50% of women considered themselves overweight, compared to 38% of men.

- 65% of the men were actually overweight, compared with 62% of the woman.

- Almost 40% of those people surveyed stated that they were on a diet.

- 60% of those surveyed were overweight, which was exactly the same percentage as last year's survey.

- More than 50% of those surveyed felt they weren't getting enough exercise.

It doesn't appear that we're getting any thinner despite all of the diet books, health clubs, fitness centers, and diet promoters! So what's the answer? Walking, of course! Walkers, by and large, are the least overweight segment of any population group. This fact has been verified in numerous medical studies.

"I Don't Really Eat That Much!"

The question I get asked most often from patients about being overweight is, "How come I keep gaining weight? I don't really eat that much." Well, the truth of the matter is that we get heavier as we get older because our physical activity tends to decrease even though our food intake stays the same. The only way to beat the battle of the bulge is to burn those unwanted pounds away. Walking actually **burns calories**. The following table will give you an idea as to the energy expended in walking, which is actually the number of calories per minute or per hour (**TABLE II**).

TABLE II

Walking Speed	Calories Burned/ Minute	Calories Burned/40 Minutes	Calories Burned/ Hour
Slow Speed (2 mph)	3-4	110-130	210-260
Moderate Speed (3 mph)	4-5	130-160	260-330
Brisk Speed (3.5 mph)	**5-6**	**235-300**	**320-380**
Fast Speed (4 mph)	6-7	190-220	380-440
Race Walking (5 mph)	7-8	220-260	440-520

A pound of body fat contains approximately 3,500 calories. When you eat 3,500 more calories than your body actually needs, it stores up that pound as body fat. If you reduce your intake by 3,500 calories, you will lose a pound. It doesn't make any difference how long it takes your body to store or burn these 3,500 calories. The result is always the same. You either gain or lose one pound of body fat, depending on how long it takes you to accumulate or burn up 3,500 calories.

You can then actually lose weight by just walking. When you walk at a speed of 3.5 mph for one hour every day, you will burn up **350 calories each day.** Therefore, if you walk for 60 minutes a day you will burn up 3,500 calories in 10 days. If you walk for 40 minutes every day you will burn up 3,500 calories in 15 days. Since there are 3,500 calories in each pound of fat, every time you burn up 3,500 calories by walking, you will lose a pound of body fat. The longer you walk, the more calories you'll burn, and that's where the Dietwalk® Plan comes into effect.

DIETWALK®: QUICK WEIGHT-LOSS PLANS

The Fit-Step: 40 Minute Plan was based on walking at a brisk pace (3.5 mph) for 40 minutes six days per week, combined with the **Diet-Step Plan: 40/40 Plan.** This weight-loss program is based upon the number of calories burned by the combination of dieting and walking. Walking at 3.5 miles per hour is a speed that can be maintained for a long duration without causing stress, strain or fatigue. We are not talking about window-shopping walking which is much too slow (1 to 2 miles/hr) and which is not at all useful in burning calories. Nor are we suggesting fast walking (4-5 miles/hr.), which is too fast to be continued for long periods of time without tiring. And we certainly are not recommending race walking (5 to 6 miles/hr), which is worthless as a permanent weight reduction plan, and has all of the same hazards and dangers that jogging has.

By following **The DIETWALK Quick Weight-Loss Walking Plans,** you will lose additional weight by actually walking off more weight, This faster weight loss occurs because you will be walking more than just the 40 minutes, 6 days/week. The following Quick Weight-Loss Plans have been designed for faster weight-loss than the weight that you lose on the Diet-Step & Fit-Step Combination Plan.

By following any one of these three Quick Weight-Loss Walking Plans, you will be able to lose more weight than you can lose on the Diet-Step/Fit-Step combination plan alone. **This additional weight-loss occurs, because you will be walking for longer periods of time every day.** Remember, it's easy to lose more weight and look your best by just walking more every day.

DIETWALK: QUICK WEIGHT-LOSS

QUICK WEIGHT-LOSS WALKING PLAN #1
Walk one hour every day and lose one additional pound every 10 days.

On this **Quick Weight-Loss Walking Plan** you can lose one additional pound every 10 days just by walking **one hour every day of the week or ½ hour twice daily**. The only difference in this plan is that you are now walking an hour every day. You will still be burning up 350 calories every hour that you walk briskly (3.5 mph).

Since it takes 10 hours of walking at 3.5 mph to burn up 3,500 calories or one pound, if you walk for an hour every day, you will **lose one additional pound every 10 days.** By following this plan you can actually **lose 3 extra pounds every month**.

QUICK WEIGHT-LOSS WALKING PLAN #2
Walk 1½ hours every day and lose one additional pound every 7 days.

For those of you who want to lose weight even faster, you can walk for **1 ½ hours every day or 45 minutes twice daily**. By walking a total of **1 ½ hours every day of the week** you will be able to speed up the walking-off-weight on this plan. When you walk 1 ½ hours every day, you will burn up 525 calories each day or 3,675 calories per week. You can see that you will lose a pound a week on this plan with a few extra (175 calories) to spare.

QUICK WEIGHT-LOSS WALKING SNACK PLAN #3
Snack on your favorite food—calorie free.

Let's say your weight is just where you'd like it to be, but you don't want to gain another ounce. Or say your weight is nowhere near what you would like it to be, but you really can't afford to gain another pound without going into another size dress. Each of you would like to be able to cheat and at least stay the same weight. Well fear no more, the **Quick Weight-Loss Walking Snack Plan** is just for you.

How about a slice of cake, French fries, a cone of ice cream, a slice of pizza, a hamburger or a glass of wine? With the **Quick Weight-Loss Walking Snack Plan** you have the perfect method that allows you to cheat without paying the price. Eat your favorite snack food, consult the following table **(TABLE III)** and walk the number of minutes listed in order to burn up the extra calories you've cheated on. The following table shows how many minutes of walking at a brisk pace (3½ mph) are necessary to burn up the caloric value of those foods listed.

If your favorite snack food is not listed on the following table, you can easily figure out the time you have to burn off your snack's calories. **Look up the number of calories of your favorite snack food and divide by the number 6.** This answer will give you the number of minutes it takes to walk off your snack. The number 6 comes from the fact that walking at a brisk pace (3.5 mph) burns approximately 6 calories per minute. Example: hamburger and roll = 438 calories. Divide 6 into 438 and you get 50. It will take you 73 minutes to walk of this snack.

TABLE III

QUICK WEIGHT-LOSS WALKING SNACK PLAN	
(Time Required to Walk Off Snacks)	
American cheese (1 slice)	16 minutes
Apple (medium)	15 minutes
Apple juice (6 oz.)	17 minutes
Bagel (1)	23 minutes
Banana (medium)	16 minutes
Beer (12 oz.)	30 minutes
Bologna sandwich	50 minutes
Candy bar (1 oz.)	45 minutes
Cake (1 slice pound)	63 minutes
Chocolate bar/nuts (1 oz.)	28 minutes
Cheese crackers (6)	35 minutes
Cheese steak (½)	55 minutes
Chicken, fried (3 pieces)	50 minutes
Chocolate cookies (3)	25 minutes
Corn chips (small pack)	33 minutes
Doughnut (jelly)	40 minutes
Frankfurter & roll	50 minutes
French fries (3 oz.)	50 minutes
Hamburger (4 oz.) and roll	73 minutes
Ice cream cone	30 minutes
Ice cream sandwich	35 minutes
Ice cream sundae	75 minutes
Milk shake, chocolate (8 oz.)	42 minutes
Muffin, blueberry	25 minutes
Orange juice (6 oz.)	16 minutes

Peanut butter crackers (6)	50 minutes
Peanuts, in shell (2 oz.)	37 minutes
Pie, apple (1 slice)	46 minutes
Pizza (1 slice)	40 minutes
Potato chips (small pack)	33 minutes
Pretzels (hard—3 small)	30 minutes
Pretzels (soft—1 Superpretzel®)	30 minutes
Shrimp cocktail (6 small)	18 minutes
Soda-cola (12 oz.)	24 minutes
Tuna fish sandwich	41 minutes
Wine, Chablis (4 oz.)	14 minutes
Whiskey, rye (1 oz.)	17 minutes

EATING AND EXERCISE

As food enters your stomach, the heart pumps a significant quantity of blood into the stomach to aid in the digestive process. This does not pose a problem when you are at rest, but if you decide to exercise immediately after eating, then there is a conflict of interests. The stomach now has to compete with the exercising muscles for the blood it needs for digestion. If the exercise gets vigorous then digestion is arrested and you begin to feel bloated and develop abdominal cramps. Exercise should therefore begin after a meal has passed through the stomach and small intestines. This takes approximately 2 hours after ingesting a large meal and from 45-60 minutes after eating a smaller meal.

Foods high in saturated fat and unhealthy fatty protein are not efficient foods for energy production and tend to store excess fat in the body's fat cells. Foods that are high in refined sugar like cakes, candy and pies can trigger an excess insulin response if they are eaten immediately before exercise. This means that the excess insulin produced as a result of the high sugar content of food, combined with the exertion of exercise, could drop the blood sugar rapidly. This could result in weakness, muscle cramps and even fainting. On the other hand foods that are higher in complex carbohydrates (whole-grain foods;

vegetable, fruits) and healthy protein (lean meats, fish, white meat of chicken and turkey; non-fat dairy products, nuts and seeds) tend to be absorbed slowly, thus avoiding the insulin spikes and the drops of blood sugar. These foods are efficient energy producers and burn calories steadily, so that no excess fat is stored in the body's fat cells.

In addition, fasting for long periods prior to exercise is in itself counterproductive. In order to replenish the energy stores (glycogen) in the liver and muscles. It is therefore necessary to eat several hours before exercising. When you fast, you deplete these energy stores, and exercise then becomes difficult and tiring without adequate fuel storage reserves for energy.

So what does this all have to do with walking and eating? Actually, not very much. Most of these rules of digestion apply to strenuous and vigorous exercise with relation to mealtime. They do, however, affect us somewhat with regards to our walking program. The most important fact to be learned from this discussion on digestive physiology is that it is essential that you don't walk immediately after eating, especially if you've consumed a relatively large meal (which you shouldn't be eating in the first place). This puts a strain on the cardiovascular system and can even deprive the heart of its own essential blood supply, particularly if you exercise vigorously immediately after eating (which you shouldn't be doing in the second place).

Walking, however, 45-60 minutes after a small to moderate meal can actually aid in digestion, by nudging the foodstuffs gently along the digestive tract. This in no way competes for the blood in the digestive tract, since your walking muscles do not require nearly as much as strenuously exercising muscles require. In fact, the gentle art of walking allows oxygen to be evenly distributed to all of the body's internal organs, which in this particular case is the digestive tract.

Recent studies indicate a three-fold advantage for dieters who walk before and after meals. As we have previously seen, walking before eating slows down our appetite-control center in the brain and makes us less hungry. Secondly, walking at any time burns calories directly as we walk. And thirdly, new studies in exercise physiology have shown that walking anywhere from 45-60 minutes after eating a small to moderate-sized meal will actually burn 10-15% more calories than walking on an empty stomach. This is explained by a term called the **thermic dynamic action of food**. What this means is that the actual digestion of food products combined with the gentle action of walking results in a higher metabolic rate, thus burning more calories per hour. Also, because of this increase in your basal metabolic rate, your body actually continues to burn more calories after you walk, than it does at rest alone.

EXERCISE INCREASES YOUR APPETITE: RIGHT? WRONG!

Another myth regarding diet and exercise is that exercise stimulates the appetite. So after you exercise you're hungry, and then you eat more, and you cancel out any calories you burned during exercise. Right? Wrong! Contrary to popular belief, walking actually decreases your appetite. It does this by several mechanisms which are described as follows:

1. **Walking burns fat rather** than carbohydrates and therefore does not drop the blood sugar precipitously. Strenuous exercises and calorie-reduction diets both drop the blood sugar rapidly, and it is this low blood sugar that stimulates your appetite and makes you hungry. Walking on the other hand is a more moderate type of exercise and consequently burns fats slowly rather than carbohydrates quickly. This results in the blood sugar remaining constant. And when the blood sugar remains level, you do not feel hungry.

2. Walking also **increases the resting basal metabolic rate (BMR).** This basal metabolic rate refers to the calories your body burns at rest in order to produce energy. When you go on a calorie restriction diet, your BMR slows up. This is because your body assumes that the reduction in calories is the result of starvation and your body wants to burn fewer calories so that you won't starve to death. The body has no way of knowing that you're on a diet. This is also one of the reasons that you don't continue to lose weight on a calorie reduction diet. The body prevents this excess weight loss by lowering its BMR, so that you stop losing weight even though you are eating the same number of calories that you ate in the beginning of your diet.

3. Walking **regulates the brain's appetite control center (appe-stat)** which controls your hunger pangs. Too little exercise causes your appetite to increase by stimulating the appestat to make you hungry. Walking, on the other hand slows the appestat down, thus decreasing your hunger pangs.

4. Walking **redirects the blood supply** away from your stomach, towards the exercising muscles. With less blood supplied to the stomach, your appetite is reduced.

5. When you combine the **Diet-Step Plan: 40 Gm Fat/ 40 Gm Fiber,** with 40 minutes of walking on the **Fit-Step: 40 Minute Walking Plan**, then the walking component powers up your basal metabolic rate, and causes you to burn more calories than if you were just following the diet alone, So, in effect, walking prevents the BMR from decreasing and burning fewer calories, as when you only diet. The result: less hunger and more calories burned when you walk every day.

6. To lose weight at an even faster rate use the DIETWALK: Quick Weight-Loss Walking plans as outlined in the beginning of this chapter.

BOOST METABOLISM TO BURN CALORIES

Some people are born with a high rate of metabolism. They essentially burn almost all of the food that they eat, and actually have difficulty gaining weight, no matter how many calories they consume. They, however, are the exception to the rule. Most of us aren't so lucky, and we have to work in order to boost our metabolic rate.

Regular exercise is the most important component in the metabolism boosting equation. The basic weight maintenance equation is: *your weight is determined by how much you eat and how much you exercise.* When you exercise regularly like a daily walking program, you take care of the movement side of the equation. This is actually the key component to preventing weight gain. By exercising more frequently you will burn calories at a faster rate, and the calorie burning will continue even after you've stopped exercising. If the exercise component of the metabolic equation is greater than the amount of food that you eat, then you will lose weight because of your increased metabolic rate. When your exercise routine is convenient and enjoyable, you'll have greater success in your exercise program. Nothing could be easier and more convenient than a regular aerobic exercise walking program. You can do it anywhere, anyplace and any time. You can walk alone or with a friend, and best of all, you do not have to join a gym to get the benefits of an aerobic exercise walking program.

Overeating and snack foods will slow down your metabolism, and cause you to gain weight. Stress, emotional eating and boredom all play a role in overeating high carbohydrate and high fat foods. If you're really hungry for snack foods, choose healthy foods to avoid excess calories, which pile on the unwanted pounds.

Overeating can be linked to one very important factor which is **portion control**. Studies have shown that overweight people who controlled their portion sizes were more likely to take weight off and keep it off permanently. Weight gain is a gradual process, and actually sneaks up on you day by day. So it's important for you to eat sensibly and avoid unhealthy snacking and be extremely mindful of portion control.

Surprisingly, there are some foods that can actually help you to boost your metabolism and burn calories. Some of these metabolism boosting foods include whole grains (including breads, cereals, pastas, legumes, beans, nuts, seeds, fresh fruits, and omega-3 fatty foods like salmon and flax seed). These foods provide a steady and constant source of fuel for your body. Your body's metabolism will then increase its calorie burning process throughout the day, and provide you with enough energy to carry on your daily functions.

Strenuous exercise after a large meal causes the increased blood supply in the stomach and intestinal tract to be diverted to the exercising muscles. This puts a strain on the cardiovascular system, especially in anyone who has a heart or circulatory problem. A calm walk, on the other hand, approximately 35-40 minutes after eating, does not stress the cardiovascular system and burns many of the excess calories that you should not have eaten in the first place. It's far better to get up and walk away from that big meal before you overstuff your face. When you physically walk away from the table you are removing yourself from temptation, but even more importantly, you are allowing the fullness control center in your brain to catch up to what's really going on in your stomach. You are actually full, but you don't know it yet. Remember, eating less and walking more are the only two ways to lose weight effectively, or, to put it another way—walk more and eat less!

WALKING BURNS BODY FAT NOT CARBOHYDRATES

If you just count calories or worse yet carbohydrates, your chances of losing weight are almost zero. Walking, however, is the only certain way towards permanent weight reduction. The majority of obese people are much less active than the majority of thin people. It is their sedentary lifestyle that accounts for their excess weight and not their overeating.

If you want to lose weight permanently, then the energy burned during your exercise should come from fats and not from carbohydrates. **During the first 35-40 minutes of moderate exercise (walking), only ⅓ of the energy burned comes from carbohydrates while ⅔ comes from body fats.** During short bursts of strenuous exercise, ⅔ of the energy burned comes from carbohydrates and only ⅓ from body fat. It stands to reason, then, that a continuous exercise like walking, which burns primarily body fats, is a lot better for permanent weight reduction than short spurts of strenuous exercise (examples: jogging, calisthenics, racquetball, etc.).

If you increase the duration of your walking from your regular daily 40 minutes to 45-60 minutes, you will burn more energy from body fats, resulting in faster weight-loss. Once you've lost your weight, you will maintain your weight better by walking 40 minutes every day than by doing calisthenics or running for 15-20 minutes. This occurs because you will be burning a higher proportion of body fats rather than carbohydrates.

PHILLY'S WALKING TIPS

A. Stay well-hydrated.

- Our bodies are composed of approximately 60% water. Water regulates almost every metabolic process. Water regulates the digestion and absorption of foods and the elimination of toxins in the bloodstream. Water also helps the blood flow to supply oxygen, energy and nutrients to every cell, tissue and organ in your body, including all of your muscles and your brain. Water also aids your metabolism in keeping your body temperature normal. If you are overheated, the body produces sweat to let you know that you need to replace the water that is lost from your body while you are perspiring.

- You can lose almost a quart of water while exercising. You should have at least a glass of water 20-30 minutes before exercise and another glass of water when you are finished with your exercise. It's a good idea to have a bottle of water with you while you're walking and you should take sips regularly while walking. Don't wait until you are thirsty. One of the very first signs of dehydration is fatigue. You can purchase water bottle safety clips that can be attached to your clothing or belt while walking. Also, on the 3 days per week that you are walking with weights, you can occasionally switch the one pound hand-held weights for two 12 ounce bottles of water in each hand. You can drink alternately from each bottle as you walk. Use the water bottles like the hand-held weights for upper body strength training exercises.

- Stay away from so-called power drinks, sodas, fruit punch, lemonade and any drinks with added sugar. A 2012 study of 810 adults published by the *American Journal of Clinical Nutrition,* reported that cutting back on liquid calories may be the quickest route to shed unwanted pounds. Participants lost more weight cutting down on liquid calories, than they did cutting down on solid calories over a period of 18 months.

The theory proposed why liquid calories are weightier than solid calories, is that people do not chew beverages, which results in a lower hormone response that signal fullness. In other words, people still are hungry after drinking sweetened beverages. Also, the sweeteners which are added to these beverages may also promote fat storage and increase your appetite.

B. Pedometer.

- Buy an inexpensive pedometer. It doesn't have to be a computer-driven model which really does nothing more than a regular pedometer. All it has to do is count your steps while you're walking. Pedometers come with an adjustable feature so that you can set your stride length into the pedometers' memory. It's easy enough to measure the length of your stride while walking by using a tape measure when you start out. Some pedometers do it automatically; others require that you set the stride length into the pedometer. The pedometer is more of a gimmick to give people something to hang their hats on while walking. If you like to use it, by all means do so. You'll be getting all of the fitness and weight loss benefits you need by walking briskly for 40 minutes, 6 days a week at approximately 3½ miles per hour whether you use a pedometer or not.

C. Efficient walking

Efficient walking will help to prevent injuries and help you to burn more calories in less time. Take the following walking Fit-Step Walking Tips:

- Relax your upper arms and shoulders as you walk.
- Walk while standing straight. Don't lean backwards or forwards.
- Take small to medium quick strides, rather than long, slow motion ones.
- Hit the ground first with your heel, and then roll your foot forward, and then push off with your toes.

- Bend your arms at an approximate 90° angle, and keep them close to the side of your body. Close your hands in loose, not tight fists.

- Swing your arms forward and backwards in rhythm with your walking stride. Keep both elbows close to your body while using your arm motion.

- Walk with your chin level to the ground. Don't look up or down. Focus on the horizon or what ever else is directly ahead of you.

D. Walking Precautions

- Avoid walking outdoors in extremely cold or hot weather, when it's very windy, or when the humidity is above 75%. Always make sure that your exercise room for indoor exercises has proper ventilation.

- In warm weather, wear breathable material that keeps your body cool. In cooler weather, layer-up your clothing to stay warm and comfortable. Socks should be padded cotton to absorb moisture. If your feet get too sweaty or you are prone to form foot blisters, then look into acrylic socks.

- Alcohol should be eliminated if you exercise, since it has an adverse effect on the heart's ability to respond to exercise. Many cases of abnormal heart rhythms have been reported from the combination of alcohol and exercise.

- Anytime you become tired, stop and rest. Don't push yourself. Walking should be fun, not work.

- Don't exercise before bedtime, since the exercise may act as a stimulant and prevent you from falling asleep.

- Avoid any exercise, including walking, immediately after eating. Time is necessary for digestion to occur.

- Your heart rate usually should not exceed 85-110 beats per minute when you are walking. A rapid heart rate is not necessary for physical fitness and good health. The target heart rate as we've seen is nothing more than a myth. If you become short of breath or tired or feel your heart pounding, stop and rest; you're probably walking too fast. If these symptoms persist or any other symptoms occur such as chest discomfort, then consult your physician immediately. Walking comfortably at approximately 3.5 miles per hour is a good speed for fitness and good health.

YOUR PHILLY FIT-STEP® DIET CHECK-UP

Even though walking is the safest and most hazard-free exercise known to men and women, it is still essential that you have a complete physical examination by your own physician before starting your walking program. It doesn't even have to be a Philly doctor. A thorough examination will usually include a complete physical examination, your personal and family medical history, a resting electrocardiogram, a chest x-ray, complete blood testing, a urinalysis or any other tests your doctor feels may be necessary. If your physician thinks that it's indicated he/she may order additional studies, like a nuclear stress electrocardiogram, an echocardiogram, a pulmonary function test or any other studies that she/he feels might be indicated.

• If any of the indoor exercises or your outdoor walking exercise causes shortness of breath, dizziness, headaches, chest pain, pain anywhere in the body or any other unusual symptoms or signs, stop immediately and consult your physician

• If you have a medical disorder that requires that you take medicine or treatment of any kind (e.g. high blood pressure, arthritis, diabetes, etc.), check with your physician before starting upon your walking program.

• Never walk if you are ill or injured. The body needs time to repair or heal itself. Wait until you are feeling better and then gradually resume your walking exercise program.

STEPS IN BUYING SHOES

1. Make sure the shoe fits properly. Shoes should be at least ½ to ¾ of an inch longer than your longest toe. The toe section should be wide and high enough so as not to cause compression of your toes.

2. The shank (section between heel and ball of foot) should be wide enough with enough cushioning material to feel comfortable and springy.

3. The upper part of the shoe should be made of materials (soft leather, fabrics, suede, etc.), which are porous and flexible.

4. The sole and heel should be made of a thick, resilient material, which absorbs the shock of walking on a hard surface. And above all, make sure the shoes are comfortable.

5. Don't choose shoes by their size. Choose them by how they fit on your feet. (Remember, sizes vary among different shoe brands and styles.)

6. The size of your feet changes as you grow older. It's a good idea to have your feet re-measured regularly.

7. In most people, one foot is larger than the other. When you go shoe shopping, have both feet measured. Then select shoes that fit the largest foot.

8. Try to find shoes that conform as closely as possible to the shape of your foot.

9. If possible, try on shoes at the end of the day: that's when your feet are their largest and widest.

10. Stand up when you are trying on shoes. Make sure there is enough space between the end of the shoe and your longest toe. "Enough space" usually means that you should have room to put your finger between the end of your longest toe and the end of the shoe.

11. Make sure the ball of your foot fits comfortably into the widest part of the shoe.

12. Don't buy shoes that feel tight, hoping they will "stretch."

13. Select shoes that fit your heel comfortably and that allow a minimum amount of slippage.

14. Walk in the shoes that you want to buy to make sure that they fit and feel right. Try the shoe on in the store, and walk around a while to make sure that the shoe feels comfortable.

15. Air cell insoles can add comfort to your feet while walking. By adding thin, extra cushioning to your walking shoes, you will walk with more spring and energy in your step. These insoles add high performance to any walking shoe.

16. Remember also, that socks can affect your shoe size, so wear the type of socks you'll be wearing while walking when you try on new walking shoes. Make sure you have a comfortable walking shoe with enough wiggle room for your toes. You also want good cushioning throughout the length of the shoe.

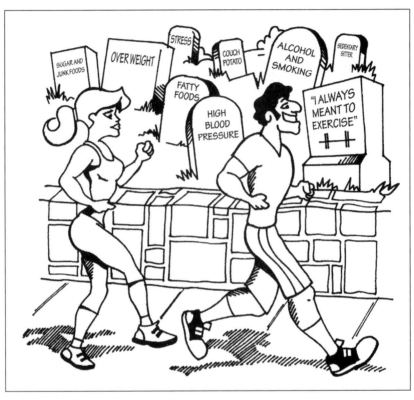

"Walking adds years to your life and life to your years."
—Dr. Walk's Diet & Fitness Newsletter

8

PHILLY'S SUPER
HEALTH WALK

"NO PAIN–NO GAIN"—FALSE!

I 've been telling my patients and readers for the past 20 years that moderate exercise promotes cardiovascular fitness and helps to prevent heart disease. Now a recent study reported from the Institute for Aerobics Research in Dallas proved that exercise doesn't have to be strenuous to be beneficial. In fact, they stated, as their major finding that, "Just a little bit of exercise is all that is needed to lower your risk of heart disease." Additional research at the Disease Control Center in Atlanta also reported that, *"Walking was as effective as any other type of exercise in preventing heart disease,* without the risk of injury or disability that occurred with strenuous exercises." They further stated that, "Over 60% of adults in the United States get little or no exercise at all." I've always contended that exercise doesn't have to be stressful, painful, or exhausting in order for it to be beneficial. In my books and in my medical practice I've always refuted the exercise enthusiasts who followed the *"no pain–no gain"* myth with reference to cardiovascular fitness. Strenuous exercise programs are actually less effective than moderate walking at 3 to 3.5 miles/hr in order to develop cardiovascular fitness and good health. And it is well documented that strenuous exercises are more likely to cause muscle, bone, and ligament injuries, aggravate high blood pressure, contribute to abnormal heart rhythms and have been known rarely cause heart attacks and strokes in people with pre-existing heart or vascular conditions.

In this same study from the Disease Control Center in Atlanta, which in fact reviewed over forty previous studies on heart disease, it was also reported that a lack of exercise by itself is as strong a risk factor for heart disease as is smoking, high blood pressure, or high blood fats. They further stated that the one statistically significant, predisposing factor in the development of heart disease that appeared in every one of the 40-plus studies was a lack of exercise, And the exercise that they cited as the most beneficial and least dangerous was a regular exercise walking program. Their research revealed that people who exercised the least had almost twice the risk of developing heart disease as those who exercised regularly.

I've also stated over and over again to my patients and in my books that the "*mythical target heart-rate zone*" is just that—a myth! No one has even proved scientifically that a rapid heart rate is essential for cardiovascular fitness. In fact, it could be potentially dangerous to keep the heart beating rapidly for a long period of time, especially in individuals who have hypertension and pre-existing heart disease. A moderate increase in your heart rate is all that is necessary to achieve maximum cardiovascular fitness.

The following findings were presented by the American Heart Association:

- Despite blood pressure, cholesterol or age, moderate exercise has an independent effect in preventing heart disease and strokes.

- Men in the lower 20% of physical fitness had a 50–60% higher incidence of developing heart disease than men who exercised regularly.

- Women in the bottom 20% zone of fitness had a 60–70% higher incidence of developing heart disease than those women who exercised regularly.

The major conclusion was that "**just a little bit more exercise**" is all that is needed to lower your risk of cardiovascular diseases. And

I think it is a bit ironic that the report ended with my long-standing quotation, *"You don't need to run a marathon in order to reduce your risk of heart disease."*

PHILLY'S SUPER FITNESS WALK

One of the most important things that you have to be aware of is that in order to begin a walking exercise program, you do not have to be an exercise fanatic. You don't need to engage in strenuous exercises or join a gym to engage in aerobic exercises or work out on weight machines. It is only necessary that you walk regularly every day. You will see that there are many ways to augment your walking program by walking at particular times of the day or evening when you would ordinarily ride. For example, when you are driving or taking the bus to work, park or get off the bus a few blocks from your place of employment, and walk that short distance. For lunch for instance, you can take a 40 minute walk. When you're at work or at home you can concentrate on using the stairs more often. For maximum aerobic conditioning, you have to walk at least 40 minutes six days a week every week. It's really not that much exercise compared to all of the benefits that you'll accrue over the month and years that follow. Walking is the single most important path that you'll take towards fitness, weight-loss, good health, and longevity.

Many people think that because they are active all day at home or in the office, they are getting adequate exercise. Nothing could be further from the truth. You are not expending the number of calories that are needed in a weight reduction or weight maintenance program by these activities. There is no doubt that you are expending energy, but you will need to supplement this with your regular walking program. Walking is a complex physiological and biomechanical process of getting from one place to another—the act of locomotion. Walking involves hundreds of muscles, thousands of nerves, and many bones, joints, and ligaments to produce a near-perfect biomechanical method of locomotion, involving the synchronous movement of the legs and arms.

The **rhythm of walking** involves a steady pace, which will become automatic, and the brain will regulate the length of your stride, your heart rate, oxygen uptake, and other physiological adjustments. You should concentrate on making smooth, even steps, avoiding spurts of speed and abrupt changes in pace. The energy expenditure over your walking period will remain constant, and your walk should leave you feeling relaxed, with effortless motion. Colon Fletcher, author of *The Complete Walker,* said it best when referring to rhythm, "An easy, unbroken rhythm can carry you along hour after hour, almost without your being aware that you are putting one foot in front of the other."

The **speed of walking** should be between 3.0 and 3.5 miles per hour, since walking is a moderate-type exercise. If you increase the speed beyond 4 miles per hour, the upper arms and shoulders swing too fast, and the lower leg muscles have to work too hard to compensate, thus producing wasteful energy expenditure. It is important that you walk at a comfortable speed, one that does not leave you breathless. This type of walking activity falls into the **aerobic** form of exercise, in which you are taking in **oxygen** as fast as you are burning it up. This is an efficient use of energy. **Anaerobic** exercise, on the other hand, is the opposite condition, which is caused by an overexertion of muscles (e.g., running fast) working beyond their capacity. This type of anaerobic exercise leads to the buildup of **lactic acid** in the muscles, causing pain, discomfort, and fatigue, a condition known as **oxygen debt**.

The **gait of walking** refers to the motions of your legs, feet, and arms during the phases of walking. Most of the energy required for walking is provided by the muscles and joints of the ankles, knees, and hips. When we over-stride or under-stride, we disrupt the natural walking gait. An easy, steady, unbroken stride will produce the rhythm and gait necessary for the effortless act of walking. Also, it is necessary to avoid toeing in or out during the walking gait, since this wastes energy. Try to concentrate on keeping your toes straight, and thus your stride will be even and rhythmic. During the act of walking, your arms swing naturally from the shoulders. Over-swinging the arms purposely during walking will reduce the efficiency of the act of walking and subsequently tire you out early during your walk. If you don't try to concentrate on the act of walking during your rhythmic stride, you will actually allow the muscles to relax and perform more efficiently.

HOW ABOUT A WALK JUST FOR FUN!

Walk whenever you can, instead of driving. If you have to drive, park somewhere a few blocks from your destination and walk the difference. Take the stairs instead of the elevator whenever possible. Take a walk when you are in a new part of town. Always walk when you are away from home to see the beauty of different surroundings. Enjoy your walk by exploring different areas around your home or office, and don't forget to look at the flowers. Take the time to smell the roses, just make sure there are no bees on them. If the weather is bad you can go to an enclosed shopping mall and walk. You can stop and look in all the windows after you've completed your regular 30-minute workout walk.

You don't have to time your pulse. You don't have to do warm up with stretching exercises before you walk. You don't have to do cool down exercises when you finish. You don't have to tire yourself or get overheated or out of breath. You don't need special clothing or equipment, just a good pair of comfortable walking shoes. You don't have to be an athlete or an acrobat. All you have to do is walk your feet for fun and you automatically, without trying, will stay fit and trim.

HOW NOT TO HAVE FUN!

Thousands of people who have joined fitness clubs in the past have been brainwashed by their so-called fitness instructors into believing the **"no pain, no gain" fallacy**. They have been intimidated into exercising "until it hurts," or when, at the point of total exhaustion, the instructor says, "Give me five more good ones. Most of these so-called fitness instructors have had very little or no training in exercise physiology, and very few, if any, have been certified or accredited by the American College of Sports Medicine.

In a recent survey of over 1500 women and men who participated in aerobic classes, over 53% sustained injuries. These injuries included strained muscles, sprained ligaments, torn cartilages, dislocated joints, stress fractures, and even slipped discs. Several cases of stress-induced strokes and heart attacks were included in this list of injuries. These injuries were sustained during strenuous aerobic exercises and calisthenics, and even low-impact aerobic exercises. Most people who engage in these exercises were not sufficiently conditioned to take the excessive strain put on their ligaments, muscles and joints. Once these injuries were sustained, the reinjury rate almost doubled because of inadequate healing time given for recovery in most cases.

HAVE YOU EVER SEEN A RUNNER SMILE?

Have you ever seen a runner smile? Of course not! It hurts too much. Runners hit the ground and impact their joints with approximately three to four times their body weight, so it is not unusual that over 60% of runners develop some form of arthritis by the time they're thirty-five to forty-five years of age. The list of potential serious injuries sustained by running and other strenuous exercises include musculo-skeletal injuries, including sprains, fractures and dislocations; compressed nerves from slipped discs and various nerve injuries; bladder and kidney injuries; menstrual irregularities and uterine and ovarian damage; heartbeat irregularities, including high blood pressure, heart attacks and strokes; exercise-induced asthma, wheezing, and partial lung collapse; stress ulcers and colon abnormalities; blood-sugar abnormalities and loss of blood minerals (calcium and potassium); heat-exhaustion and heat-stroke; decreased sex-drive and infertility; retinal detachments and eye hemorrhages; anemia and other blood abnormalities; and finally, anxiety, depression and obsessive-compulsive behavior (running mania). *It certainly doesn't sound like they're having fun, does it?*

Walking is kinder to your body and produces better health, fitness and weight-control benefits than jogging or other strenuous exercises without the stress, pain, and strain on your body. Medical research has proven again and again that exercise does not have to be painful in order to have beneficial results. The so-called "no pain–no gain" theory is actually insane. Walking is the only exercise that you can safely continue for the rest of your life for a healthier, happier you. *Walking certainly is the road to fitness and fun.*

WALKING AROUND KEEPS BLOOD SUGAR DOWN

Walking in most cases enables Type I diabetics (insulin dependent), to reduce their insulin requirements by approximately 35%, and Type II diabetics (non-insulin dependent) to reduce their oral medication dosages by approximately 50-75% and in some cases to eliminate medication entirely. This occurs because walking not only burns calories including sugar, but walking increases the cells' sensitivity to insulin. Type I diabetics therefore need less injections of insulin, and Type II diabetics become more sensitive to the production of their own body's insulin and require less oral medication.

Once the insulin or oral medication doses are reduced, the diabetic's cardiovascular risk factors improve. A diabetic normally has increased risk factors for heart attacks and strokes. Walking appears to reduce these risk factors by controlling blood sugar, decreasing serum cholesterol, making the blood less likely to clot, reducing total body weight, and by opening the tiny capillaries that feed blood to the extremities, organs, tissues, cells, and to the heart muscle itself. An exercise program for the diabetic requires careful medical supervision. Medication dosages (insulin or pills) should never be changed without a physician's approval.

In general, strenuous exercise should be avoided because it may accelerate sugar absorption which could result in sudden hypoglycemia (low blood sugar) and could result in fainting spells or other serious complications. This is particularly true if a diabetic attempts to exercise too soon after a meal. At least 60-90 minutes should elapse before a diabetic begins exercising. The beauty of a walking program is that it is a moderate aerobic-type of exercise without any of the hazards of strenuous exercise. This is especially important in the diabetic, since he or she is particularly vulnerable to the side effects of strenuous exercise.

Walking avoids the sudden drops in blood sugar that so often accompany strenuous exercise. Walking eliminates the high-impact stress on the extremities' nerve-endings and blood vessels, which are particularly subject in the diabetic to injury from high-impact sports.

Walking gently burns calories, thus lowering blood sugar moderately. This enables the diabetic to eventually lower his or her dosage of insulin or oral medication, after the body gradually adjusts to the wonderful world of walking. *Walking keeps your feet on the ground and your blood sugar down.*

WALKING FIGHTS OBESITY

In the majority of cases, obesity results from too little exercise and too much fat in the diet. Many medical studies have shown that excess weight causes cardiovascular disease with increased mortality. These same studies also reveal that life expectancy improves following weight reduction. Obese people have a significantly higher incidence of hypertension than non-obese persons. The excess body weight demands a higher cardiac output (pumping out blood) to meet the increased metabolism of an overweight person's body. This in turn causes the left chamber of the heart to gradually enlarge because of this extra workload. The combined effect of obesity, hypertension, and heart enlargement may eventually lead to heart failure and death. A low-fat, high-fiber diet combined with walking can help to lower the blood pressure and the complications that occur from obesity and hypertension.

Being obese causes an alteration in the body's chemistry and metabolism. The blood sugar goes up dramatically, with obesity often leading to the development of diabetes. The uric acid in the blood becomes elevated, often leading to kidney stones and attacks of gout. Obese people have higher levels of triglycerides (sugar fats) and the "bad" LDL-cholesterol in their blood. They also have lower blood levels of the "good" HDL-cholesterol. These altered blood fats will eventually lead to heart and vascular disease. These abnormal blood chemistries can be reversed to normal levels, if weight reduction occurs before permanent complications result. The Framingham Heart Study has recently reported that "Obesity just by itself has been listed as an independent risk factor for coronary heart disease." This study stated that obesity just by itself was enough to cause a significant increase in the risk of coronary heart disease and premature death in both men and women.

The Philly Fit-Step Walking Diet is the way to win the war against obesity:

- **Diet-Step®: Plan**: Diet consisting of 40 Grams Fat/ 40 Grams Fiber daily.

- **Fit-Step® Plan**: Aerobic exercise walking plan, 40 minutes, six days per week. Or divide your walk into two 20 minute sessions daily.

- **Power Body-Shaping Plan**: Aerobic exercise walking program for 40 minutes, six days per week, with the addition of walking with hand-held weights for 40 minutes, 3 days per week. Again two 20 minute sessions daily works just as well. This plan builds strong bones and muscles and effectively reduces your weight, including your blood fats, and therefore reduces your risk of cardiovascular and cerebrovascular disease and early death.

WALK AWAY FROM TYPE A

Emotional stress can precipitate heart attacks in both women and men with no known history of coronary artery disease. Type A behavior (high-strung, aggressive personalities) has also been associated with an increased incidence of coronary heart disease, completely independent of other coronary risk factors. And patients who already had coronary heart disease with Type A behavior were shown to have more severe artery involvement than did patients with heart disease that had Type B behavior (non-aggressive, more relaxed type personalities). In today's corporate America, fast paced executives with Type A personalities can be found just as often in women as in men. By climbing the corporate ladder, women and men have also climbed into a high-risk category for strokes and heart attacks. Women also have the added stress of juggling work and home responsibilities. What we all need to do is make time for ourselves to relax. Instead of spending all of that time in front of your computer, go out and take a nice refreshing, oxygen-filled walk.

New research has demonstrated that emotional stress can cause coronary disease as well as aggravate it in patients who already have heart disease. And all of these studies also show that by reducing

stress, coronary heart disease and hypertension can often be prevented in normal patients and controlled in patients who already have
heart or blood pressure problems. Type A behavior can be modified
with stress management techniques. These techniques include personal counseling, avoiding stressful situations, and our true-blue, loyal
friend—*walking*. Walking has been proven over and over again to significantly reduce stress and tension, alleviate anger and hostility, decrease fatigue and malaise, and control anxiety and depression. **Walk
away from stress today and your heart will be O.K.**

WALK AWAY FROM HIGH BLOOD PRESSURE

According to the American Heart Association, more than one out
of every four people in the United States has high blood pressure, and
the incidence is higher in women than it is in men. Among people
age 65 years and older, approximately two out of three people suffer
from hypertension. There are approximately 57.7 million Americans
who have high blood pressure according to the Heart Association
Council for High Blood Pressure Research. Many of these people are
at considerable risk for developing strokes, heart attacks, heart failure
and kidney disease, unless they receive medical treatment. Women
are particularly vulnerable to the complications of hypertension.
Unfortunately, most people with high blood pressure have no symptoms and may have hypertension for many years before it is diagnosed. Remember, always get your blood pressure checked regularly.

Many cases of mild hypertension can be controlled without the use
of medication. These methods include weight reduction, salt restriction, cessation of smoking, alcohol restriction, decreasing saturated
fats and cholesterol in the diet, stress reduction and exercise. It should
be pointed out that the majority of studies on the benefits of exercise
for lowering blood pressure have used *walking* as the best moderate
intensity exercise for this purpose. Jogging and other strenuous exercises can actually raise blood pressure during the actual exercise.

Two major studies reported in a recent issue of the *Journal of the
American Medical Association* proved without a doubt that regular
exercise, particularly walking, can decrease the risk of developing

heart disease and high blood pressure by more than 50 percent. The first report studied over 6,000 women and men who had no previous history of high blood pressure. Over a period of 4 years, people who did not exercise regularly ran a 52 percent higher risk of developing hypertension. The second study followed 17,000 women and men over a period of 16 years. Those who exercised regularly experienced only one-half the death rate from heart disease and hypertension. This study showed lower blood pressures and lower death rates, particularly in women who walked regularly.

There are several physiological mechanisms responsible for the blood pressure lowering effect of exercise. They include improved cardiac output of blood, decreased peripheral vascular resistance to the flow of blood, slower pulse rate, dilation of small arteries, thinning of the blood and a reduced release of *catecholamines* and *angiotensin* (the hormones that cause high blood pressure). The fact remains, however, that no matter what the physiological reasons are, walking lowers your blood pressure. All you have to remember is that if you *keep your feet on the ground, you'll keep your blood pressure down!*

BEAT THE ODDS AGAINST HEART DISEASE

Coronary heart disease is responsible for over one-half million deaths each year in the United States. It causes more deaths each year than all forms of cancer combined. There are over 5½ million women and men who have been diagnosed as having coronary artery disease. It is estimated that there are at least 2½ million other Americans with undiagnosed coronary heart disease, many of them under the age of 50. It has also recently been shown that pre-menopausal women are also at risk for heart disease. The misconception was that only post-menopausal women were at risk because of their lack of estrogen.

Coronary artery disease is caused by the build-up of fat deposits in the arteries (atherosclerosis). This disease begins slowly, early in life, and usually doesn't produce symptoms until middle age. This build-up of fat in the arteries, also known as plaque, is of particular importance in women whose coronary arteries have a smaller diameter than the coronary arteries in men. Unfortunately, this condition often goes undetected until the individual has her first heart attack, which may in fact be fatal. Although we have made great strides in the treatment of heart attacks, the emphasis must rest on preventing this slowly progressive disease (atherosclerosis) from occurring. It is estimated that more than 60 billion dollars are spent each year in the treatment of coronary heart disease and less than a million dollars yearly are spent on the prevention of this disease.

In order to prevent or slow the progress of atherosclerosis we must be aware of the 10 *risk factors* which contribute to the development of this disease. One risk factor that we can't control is heredity; however, those people who have a strong family history of heart disease should pay particular attention to the risk factors that we can modify. The 9 risk factors which we can control ourselves or with medical treatment include: **cigarette smoking, excess alcohol consumption, excess caffeine, obesity, high blood pressure, high blood cholesterol, diabetes, stress** and **inactivity**.

One risk factor increases your risk of a heart attack by 25%. If you have two of these risk factors, it increases your likelihood of getting a heart attack by 35%. Three will increase your chances by 45% and four will increase your risk by 55-60%. How would you like to be able to eliminate or reduce almost all of these risk factors in one fell swoop? There is no need to worry about these risk factors if you start walking like your life depended on it. Believe me, it does! **Walking** can actually help you remove or reduce these risk factors to a minimum with a little additional help from your willpower.

How is this possible? The body that exercises doesn't want or need to *smoke* or drink *alcohol* or *caffeine*. The person who walks stays at his or her *ideal weight*. Walking lowers your *blood pressure* and your *blood cholesterol*. If you're a *diabetic* or have diabetic tendencies, walking helps to improve and regulate sugar metabolism. Walking is a sure fire method to ward off the evils of *stress* and *tension*. And, finally, walking every day completely eliminates the coronary risk factor of *inactivity*. When you do the Philly Fit-Step Walking Diet, you are beating the odds against all 9 risk factors of heart disease.

DON'T STROKE OUT!

Strokes are the third leading cause of deaths in the United States each year. The most frequent contributing factor is high blood pressure. Approximately 65% of all strokes occur in people who never knew they had high blood pressure or in people who had hypertension but did not take their medication regularly.

High blood pressure speeds up the process of atherosclerosis ("hardening of the arteries"). Untreated hypertension damages the lining walls of the arteries and allows fatty deposits to collect in the arteries. This in turn sets the stage for blood clots to form in the blood vessels of the brain, which can cause a stroke. High blood pressure also can weaken the walls of the blood vessels of some predisposed individuals, so that a balloon or aneurysm forms. The combination of high blood pressure and extreme physical exertion (example: jogging, weight-lifting, etc.) may cause this aneurysm to rupture, which results in a hemorrhage into the brain producing another form of stroke.

Fortunately, stroke-related deaths have declined by almost 45% in the United States in the past 10 years. This is due primarily to the widespread, successful treatment of high blood pressure. People are beginning to realize that they have to continue taking their high blood pressure medicine indefinitely, in order to prevent strokes from occurring.

Stopping smoking also is important in preventing strokes from occurring. The carbon monoxide from smoking damages the blood vessel walls, and speeds up the process of atherosclerosis. The early treatment of diabetes and obesity also helps to slow down this process of hardening of the arteries, which leads to hypertension and stroke. Also reducing salt and stress helps to lower blood pressure and in turn reduces your risk of stroke.

According to most medical authorities, a moderate program of regular exercise is extremely important in controlling high blood pressure and in preventing strokes. You heard it—**moderate exercise!** Walking is the exercise most often prescribed by physicians to control hypertension. Walking actually lowers your blood pressure and can help to prevent strokes and heart attacks.

EXERCISE AND BRAIN POWER

In a recent study in the *Annals of Internal Medicine (Annals Internal Medicine.* 2006:144:73-81, 135-136), it was reported that regular exercise may delay the onset of dementia. This study showed that a moderate amount of exercise could in fact reduce a person's risk of dementia by almost 40%. Over a six year period, 1,750 adults aged 65 and older without cognitive impairment, were included in this study. The participants reported their exercise patterns at two year intervals, which included walking, swimming, hiking, calisthenics, water aerobics, stretching, weight training, or a combination of one or more of these activities.

The rate of dementia was 13.0 per 1,000 participants who exercised three times a week versus 19.7 per 1,000 participants who exercised fewer than three times per week. The group that benefited the most were people who were the frailest at the start of the study. This finding was interpreted that older people should "use it even after you start to lose it," because exercise may slow the progression of age-related diseases, including dementia. Earlier studies have reported conflicting results on the relationship between physical activity and dementia. This is the first study to demonstrate a real correlation between the level of physical activity and brain function including the risk for developing dementia.

This study stated that the current recommendations for all adults including the elderly, should include at least 60 minutes daily of a moderate-intensity exercise to promote good health and to decrease the risk for chronic diseases and early death. They further point out that these exercise recommendations may help to prevent cognitive decline and neurodegenerative diseases in the elderly.

Walking, which is by far the best moderate aerobic exercise, combined with strength training weight baring exercises, appears to be the best combination for improving physical fitness and preventing senile dementia and/or Alzheimer's disease. Swimming and water aerobics are also good alternatives or additions to a walking program for a successful exercise program.

EXERCISE AND ARTERIES

A study at the University of Pennsylvania showed increased blood flow into the body's arteries in patients who exercised regularly. This was apparently due to the fact that the exercise helped to keep the arteries open by decreasing the amount of inflammation inside the walls of the arteries. This inflammatory process which occurs in your arteries is a natural process of aging. The inflammation which occurs in your blood vessels causes the blood vessel vault to swell, depositing cholesterol plaques on the artery walls which in turn narrows the opening through which your blood flows. This decreased blood flow can be the cause of the heart attack, stroke or blood clot.

Inflammation can make the joints swell in patients who have arthritis. Doctors often give cortisone to patients with arthritis to reduce the amount of inflammation in the joints. Exercise acts like cortisone by helping to decrease the inflammation that occurs in the arthritic patient's joints as well as the inflammation that occurs in patient's arteries that are prone to cardiovascular disease. This exercise does not have to be strenuous. Moderate exercise like walking helps to keep the arteries opened by decreasing the amount of inflammation inside the walls of the blood vessels. In fact, it has been shown in repeated studies that moderate exercise helps to reduce the inflammatory process in the arteries significantly more than strenuous exercise which can in itself cause more inflammation in your body's arteries.

WALK OFF WEIGHT & DEPRESSION

According to a recent study, overweight women who stayed at home had a significant increase in the incidence of depression. It was further found that both of these conditions can be alleviated by participating in a regular walking program. This study found that overweight women ages 25-35 who stayed at home have experienced significantly more depression than their peers who work outside the home, possibly secondary to the lack of socialization and/or intellectual stimulation. These findings are in agreement with several other studies that have shown a positive association between exercise and mood.

The women in this study were between the ages of 20-40 years, and were considered moderately to severely overweight. They all exhibited complaints of mild to moderate depression. The women were randomized into a walking group and a control group who did not walk. The walking group walked 45 minutes daily, five days per week, for a period of 12 weeks. The control group did not engage in any physical exercise program whatsoever. Compared to the control group, the women who walked regularly lost weight and felt less depressed.

The results confirm studies that physical exercise, especially a moderate walking program, is a plausible treatment for mild to moderate depression, particularly in overweight women, who were stay-at-home mothers or whose jobs involved at-home duties. This walking program can act as an alternative to medication in women who prefer nonpharmacological treatment for depression, or as an adjunct to antidepressant medication. The fact that these women lost weight was a significant factor in improving the level of depression.

Walking, as we have seen, improves mood and has a natural antidepressant and a natural appetite-suppressant effect by increasing the brain's endorphin levels and by decreasing the brain's appetite control mechanism (the appestat). A regular walking program also produces continuous infusion of oxygen to the body's cells and also rids the body of toxins, particularly free radicals, which tend to cause degenerative changes in the body. These free radicals can not only physically alter the brain cells and cause depression, they can also cause the appetite-suppressing mechanism in the brain to be faulty and increase the level of hunger, causing obesity.

Walking women, by and large, are less depressed and less overweight, whether they are stay-at-home moms, working stay-at-home jobs, or even women who work outside the home. Walking women win the fight against obesity and depression.

A DAILY WALK KEEPS ARTHRITIS AWAY

Recent research suggests that walking may be the best exercise for most forms of arthritis. Most people with arthritis can benefit from a regular exercise program according to the majority of rheumatologists. And the exercise that most of the doctors recommended for their patients with arthritis was walking. Walking strengthens the muscles and ligaments that are attached to the arthritic joints. This helps to relieve the pain that occurs when the bones rub against each other. Walking also may prevent some of the joint inflammation and deformity that is associated with arthritis. The gentle joint motions of walking may relieve joint pain and swelling. Just make sure that you take it easy and rest frequently. Don't walk through pain.

The recurrent pain and joint swelling associated with arthritis acts as a depressant in the majority of patients with arthritis. Depression in turn leads to lethargy and inactivity. The inactivity instead of relieving the pain in most arthritics tends to lead to more joint involvement and greater immobility. Walking on the other hand with its biochemical and psychological mood-elevating effects, acts as a natural antidepressant in the arthritic patient. Walking does wonders to improve the arthritic's feeling of well-being and it improves the vicious cycle of pain, depression, and subsequent immobility.

Any patient who has some form of arthritis must be monitored closely by his or her personal physician. Each patient is an individual and will respond differently to various forms of exercise. Just as complete inactivity may lead to a worsening of arthritis, too much activity, especially strenuous exercises, may also have an adverse effect on arthritis. Listen to the advice of your own physician. Most doctors, however, will recommend a graduated walking program for the majority of their patients. **Don't let pain keep you in. Get out there and Walk to Win!**

WALKING AND COLON CANCER

A recent study at the State University of New York in Buffalo has now linked even colon cancer to lack of physical activity. This condition had been previously thought to be caused only by a *low-fiber, high-fat diet.* Now, however, it appears that men with sedentary jobs (bus drivers, bookkeepers, accountants, computer operators, etc.) are 60 percent more likely to get cancer of the colon compared to more physically active men (longshoremen, mailmen, and mechanics, etc.).

In this study, the occupations of approximately 500 rectal and colon cancer patients were compared to the occupations of over 1,400 patients with other diseases. Women who had spent more that 20 years in completely sedentary jobs had twice the incidence of colon cancer as compared to those women with active jobs. And women who worked at low-activity jobs had 1½ times the risk of colon cancer as active workers.

Physical activity, especially a regular *walking program,* appears to stimulate the movement of waste products through the colon, thus decreasing the time that the potential waste carcinogens are in contact with the wall of the colon. This is a similar theory to that which explains why a high-fiber, low-fat diet also helps to prevent colon cancer.

EXERCISE DECREASES RISK OF BREAST & UTERINE CANCER

In a study from Harvard School of Public Health, it was found that women who began exercising and playing sports as young girls appear to develop body changes that reduce their risk of developing breast and uterine cancers. These findings were based on the facts that exercise in young girls delays the onset of menstruation by several years. The early onset of menstruation is considered to be a potential risk factor for developing breast and uterine cancers. Active young women who engaged in sports were also noted to have fewer and lighter menstrual periods, which usually reduces the production of female hormones. This fact may be responsible for the decreased risk of developing both breast and uterine cancers in active young women.

Women who continue their exercise program into later life have less body fat and more lean muscle mass. These women also tend to eat a low-fat diet throughout their adult years. It is a known fact that excess saturated fat in the diet produces excess amounts of estrogen, which increases the risk of breast cancer. In this particular study of over 5000 women, it was also found that the leaner active women produced not only less estrogen but a less potent form of estrogen than did inactive obese women. This less potent form of estrogen was less likely to cause breast and uterine cancer as was the more potent form of estrogen produced by overweight women. These findings showed that sedentary women had a 2½ times greater risk of developing cancer of the uterus and twice the risk of developing breast cancer.

Prostate Cancer Patients Do Better With Exercise

New research suggests that exercise may be a universal supplement to the treatment of prostate cancer. The authors of a report published in the January 2011 issue of the *Journal of Clinical Oncology* used a research database and tracked the health habits of 2,705 patients who were diagnosed with prostate cancer over a period of 18 years. The researchers found that all sorts of physical activity after the diagnosis was made reduced overall mortality. This finding was independent of whatever type of prostate cancer treatment that these patients had previously received for their disease.

This report showed that men who walked for 90 minutes or more per week had a 46% lower risk of death from all causes compared with men who walked less than 90 minutes weekly. It was also found that those men who exercised vigorously for three hours or more per week had a 49% lower risk of overall mortality and a 61% lower risk of dying from prostate cancer, compared with men who had exercised for less than one hour per week. This report also showed that men who had exercised both before and after their diagnosis was made did even better than those men who had only started exercising after they were diagnosed with prostate cancer.

FITNESS IN ADOLESCENTS AND YOUNG ADULTS

A recent article in the *Journal of the American Medical Association* (*JAMA*, December 21, 2005, Vol. 294, No. 23, 2981-2988) showed that both adolescents and young adults with poor cardio-respiratory fitness were at considerable risk for developing cardiovascular disease. There is strong evidence that a low level of physical activity is associated with a higher morbidity and mortality from all causes including cardiovascular disease and cancer. Population studies show that physical activity levels are extremely low in the United States, particularly in adolescents and young adults.

This study showed that adolescents and adults with low levels of fitness were two to four times more likely to be overweight than were participants who exercised regularly. Both adolescents and adults who were less fit were more likely to have high blood pressure and high cholesterol. There was also shown to be a relationship between low fitness levels and the incidence of the "metabolic syndrome," which consists of a combination of high blood pressure, high blood fats, obesity, and diabetes or insulin intolerance.

This report indicated that the low fitness levels in both adolescents and adults are an important and prevalent public health problem in the United States. This correlation between low fitness levels and cardiovascular risk gives rise to a potential trend of increasing mortality and morbidity from chronic diseases caused by obesity and inactivity.

Although adolescents are not usually considered at short-term risk for developing cardiovascular disease, they develop risk factors during adolescence and young adulthood, which sets the stage for heart disease in middle and older age. There is little doubt that adolescents who are unfit and overweight are at considerable risk for developing cardiovascular disease as they age. Many studies in adult men and women report an association between low levels of physical activity and increased mortality from cardiovascular disease and other disorders including cancer.

It has been further shown that a regular exercise program started at any age will improve fitness and will lower the risk of developing cardiovascular disease and other degenerative diseases of aging. In order to prevent this epidemic of obesity and inactivity in adolescents and young adults from occurring, an education campaign needs to be implemented in the schools and in the work place in order to reverse these negative health behaviors. These individuals need to be educated as to the health benefits of physical activity, which is necessary to improve cardiovascular fitness and prevent this epidemic of obesity from occurring in young adults and adolescents.

YES, WOMEN ARE REALLY DIFFERENT FROM MEN!

"Yes, Women Are Different From Men" was the first page headline in a recent edition of *The Medical Tribune*. Finally, new research has discovered that there are significant differences in the physiology of women and men. These differences extend far beyond the obvious reproductive biological differences. These differences affect almost every organ system in the body, including the heart, brain, digestive tract, nervous system, and even the skin.

With reference to the heart, women's hearts beat faster at rest than do men's hearts. Also, the electrical behavior of the conducting tissue in the heart is different in women and men which may explain the normal difference in the EKGs of women and men. It has previously been found that a woman's coronary arteries are smaller than those of a man. These factors have to be taken into consideration in the diagnosis, treatment, and prevention of heart disease in women. Physicians are just recognizing the difference in treating women with coronary artery disease, since they often present with different symptoms than men when they are having a heart attack.

A long held fallacy in medicine has been that whatever research was done on male patients, for example, physiology and reactions to different medications, could be interpreted as being the same for women. Nothing could be further from the truth. For example, women metabolize different medications differently from men, which must be taken into careful consideration when treating female patients. Many diseases and medications affect women differently and these differences must be considered when formulating different types of treatments for various diseases. Yes, women are really different from men, and it's about time that the medical establishment is becoming aware of that important difference.

Many of these differences in physiology may explain the difference in the fitness response to exercise in women. The *maximum oxygen uptake* is defined as the highest rate at which oxygen can be taken up from the atmosphere and utilized by the body during exercise. It is frequently used to indicate the cardio-respiratory fitness of an individual. Even though men have a larger overall muscle mass than women, women have more long-term endurance capacity. This may in part be explained by a woman's ability to sustain her maximum oxygen uptake longer by steady, consistent exercise.

Men, on the other hand, frequently engage in short bursts of energy expenditure like jogging, racquetball, strenuous weight lifting, etc. This type of strenuous activity does not increase the maximum uptake capacity (uptake and distribution of oxygen throughout the body) for a long enough time to develop maximum aerobic fitness. Women, on the other hand, develop aerobic fitness more slowly than men; however, their fitness and endurance levels are more consistent and long lasting. In many cases, women who engage in moderate exercise activity like walking, stationary bike, treadmill, etc. are more likely to stay aerobically fit than if they engaged in strenuous exercises. However, both men and women can achieve maximum cardiovascular fitness, weight reduction and good health on the Philly Fit-Step Walking Diet.

WALKING COMPARABLE TO VIGOROUS EXERCISE IN REDUCING WOMEN'S CARDIOVASCULAR RISK

As reported recently in the *The New England Journal of Medicine*, postmenopausal women who walk regularly lowered their heart disease risk just as much as women who do more vigorous exercise, such as jogging or playing sports. This study is documented evidence that regular walking can prevent heart attacks in women.

The study included over 70,000 women between the ages of 50 and 79, who were asked about the types of physical activity that they engaged in each week. None of the women included in the study had previous evidence of cardiovascular disease at the beginning of the study. During the follow-up period of 3 years, only 345 women developed heart disease.

Women who either walked regularly or vigorously exercised regularly were less likely than sedentary women to develop cardiovascular disease, and both types of exercise were associated with the same risk reduction. Women who spent at least 2½ hours per week walking briskly or engaging in vigorous exercise were each 30% less likely than others to develop heart disease.

This study also concluded that prolonged sitting appeared to counteract the benefits of any type of exercise and women who spent more time sitting were more likely than others to develop cardiovascular disease.

WALKING IMPROVES BRAIN FUNCTION

Women who walk regularly are less likely to experience memory loss and other brain function declines that can be associated with aging. These findings were presented at a recent meeting of the American Academy of Neurology. This research entailed the study of approximately 6000 women ages 65 and older. All of these women were given cognitive function testing at the beginning of the study and again after eight years. Women who walked the most demonstrated less memory loss than those in the lower exercise groups, even after adjusting for age and other coexisting medical conditions.

Researchers feel that there is a significant correlation between physical activity and chemical activity in the brain. As we saw in the previous study on depression, exercise has the ability to increase the availability of certain brain neurotransmitters (serotonin) and mood-elevating brain chemicals (beta-endorphins). There can be little doubt then, that women who walk regularly have better brain function as they age.

TAKE A HAPPY WALK

Americans are walking again like never before. According to the President's Council on Physical Fitness report, walking is the single most popular adult exercise in America. With over 52 million adherents, the numbers are steadily increasing as men and women of all ages are walking for health, fitness and fun. Walking is an exercise whose time has finally come. Why not? It's easy, safe, fun, and it makes you feel and look great.

According to the latest Roper Poll, over 50% of Philadelphians stated that walking was their favorite form of exercise. That's about the same percentage as most cities across the nation. Surprised? Don't be. The fitness industry would like us to think otherwise. That's why hundreds of millions of dollars are spent each year on advertising health and fitness clubs, jogging apparel, aerobic centers, fitness machines and any other gimmicks that these advertisers can use to empty your wallets. Well, take heart America, they can fool some of the people some of the time, but not all of the people all of the time. Fitness centers and gyms won't advertise walking because they can't make a dime from it.

Walking is something that two people, no matter how different their physical conditions, can do together. It is a companionable exercise in which you enjoy each other's company and at the same time get all the benefits of exercising. Walking is a great escape. You can get away from the phone, from the office, or from home for a little while, and take that needed time to relax. You can walk to think out a problem or walk to forget one. Walking acts as a tranquilizer to help us relax and it can work as a stimulant to give us energy. The late famous cardiologist Dr. Paul Dudley White said, "A *vigorous 3 mile walk will do more good for an unhappy but otherwise healthy adult than all the medicine and psychology in the world.*" Don't make the common mistake of thinking that walking is too easy to be a good exercise. On the contrary, walking is not only the safest, but it's the best exercise in the world. If you're overweight, then walking is your best choice since you won't be putting excessive stress on the ligaments, muscles, and joints.

How you walk also tells whether you're happy, sad, angry, ambitious or just plain lazy. Walkers with a long stride, a greater arm swing, and a bounce to their step are happy, ambitious and self-assured, whereas walkers with a short stride, foot shuffle or drag and a short arm swing are often depressed, unhappy and angry. Recent studies in women indicate that arm swing is the most indicative factor of their mood. The greater the arm swing, the happier, more vigorous and less depressed a person is. A short arm swing indicated that a person was angry, frustrated and unhappy. Stretch out your stride, swing your arms, and put a bounce in your step whenever and wherever you walk. That's your road to good health, a successful career and a long, happy life. Believe it! It works!

WONDERFUL WORLD OF WALKING

There is considerable agreement among most exercise physiologists that exercise on a moderate, steady basis has a tranquilizing effect. A rhythmic exercise like walking for 40 minutes seems to be the most effective method for producing this tranquilizing effect. Several theories have been proposed to explain this tranquilizing effect. One current theory is that a slight increase in body temperature affects the brainstem and results in a rhythmic electrical activity in the cortex of the brain. This produces a more relaxed state and is the direct result of exercise. Other studies indicate that there is an increase in brain chemicals, particularly a group of chemicals called the endorphins. These appear to have a tranquilizing or sedative effect and result in relaxation.

In a recent study reported in the *New England Journal of Medicine,* researchers suggested that regular exercise may increase the secretion of two chemicals called *beta-endorphin* and *beta-lipotropin.* These substances act as chemical painkillers or tranquilizers and thus can influence the body's metabolism and give a sense of tranquility and well-being. This study noted that with exercise, these levels of chemicals increased, and with more strenuous exercise, this increase was even greater. This may, in part, explain the "runners' high" or the feeling of euphoria that is reported with high-intensity exercise. They stated that this also might explain the frequency with which runners sustain fractured bones while running without feeling any pain.

Walking, on the other hand, produces only a moderate rise in these brain chemicals. This results in a relaxed state of mind and produces a tranquilizing effect on the entire nervous system. Since walking is not a strenuous exercise, the level of these brain chemicals does not go too high, thus avoiding the analgesic or pain-killing effect produced with high-intensity exercises. This enables the walker to be aware of any type of pain, for example if she or he turns his or her ankle or foot while walking. The runner, on the other hand, because of the high euphoric-analgesic levels of these brain chemicals, may not actually feel any type of pain, for example, chest pain from a heart attack, and he/she may suffer a coronary without being aware of the pain. The abnormally high levels of these brain chemicals in this particular case are another example of too much of a good thing.

The wonderful world of walking witchcraft is just the potion you need to combat everyday stress and tension. The calm, serene enchantment of walking alleviates tension, nervousness, anxiety and stress. Let the wonderful world of walking lead you down the peaceful path of restful relaxation.

BENEFITS OF PHILLY'S SUPER HEALTH WALK

- Walking decreases the risk of hypertension and all of its cardiovascular complications.

- Walking decreases the risk of vascular diseases, such as strokes and heart attacks

- Walking decreases the risk of developing adult-onset type II diabetes, with its subsequent complications, such as eye disorders and vascular diseases.

- Walking also reduces blood sugar levels and lowers the risk of obesity, diabetes, and heart disease.

- Walking has been shown to be helpful in decreasing anxiety and depression. Also walking enhances mood and mental well-being.

- Walking also helps to prevent several degenerative neurological diseases, such as Alzheimer's disease and degenerative joint diseases, such as arthritis.

- Walking decreases the risk of many types of cancer, including colon, prostate, and breast cancer.

- Walking increases bone density and reduces the risk of osteoporosis.

- Walking makes you feel and actually look younger.

- Walking adds years to your life and life to your years.

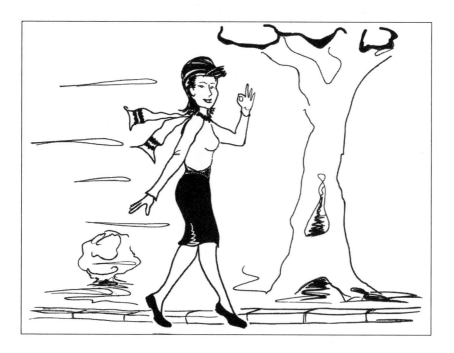

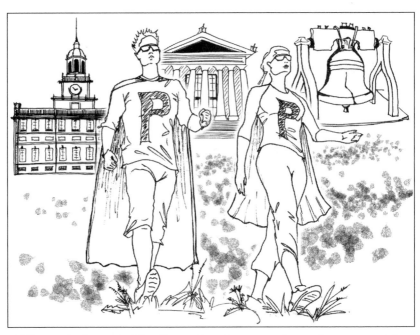

"Our mission on this planet is to reverse the aging process in these sedentary earthlings by getting them to walk every day. Let's start in this city called Philadelphia."

9

LOOK YOUNGER & LIVE LONGER

OXYGEN: THE VITAL INGREDIENT

With the advent of the computer age, most people are forced by design to do less and less physical labor. It would seem logical that this would result in more energy being available for other activities. However, how many times have you noticed that the less you do, the more tired you feel, whereas the more active you are, the more energy you have for other activities? Exercise improves the efficiency of the lungs, the heart and the circulatory system in their ability to take in and deliver oxygen throughout the entire body. This oxygen is the catalyst which burns the fuel (food) we take in to produce energy. Consequently, the more oxygen we take in, the more energy we have for all of our activities.

Oxygen is the vital ingredient that is necessary for our survival. Since oxygen can't be stored, our cells need a continuous supply in order to remain healthy. Walking increases your body's ability to extract oxygen from the air, so that increased amounts of oxygen are available for every organ, tissue and cell in the body. Walking actually increases the total volume of blood, making more red blood cells available to carry oxygen and nutrition to the tissues, and to remove carbon dioxide and waste products from the body's cells. This increased saturation of the tissues with oxygen is also aided by the opening of small blood vessels, which is another direct result of walking.

193

So let's take that first step for energy, fitness and pep. Walking every day will keep a fresh supply of oxygen surging through your blood vessels to all of your body's hungry cells. Don't disappoint these little fellows because you depend on them as much as they depend on you. If you short-change them on their daily oxygen supply, they'll take it out on you in the form of illness and disease. The Philly Fit-Step Walking Diet helps to keeps the doctor away.

OUR BODIES ARE MADE FOR WALKING

People don't always behave in their own best interests and that includes any type of exercise including walking. A recent survey showed that 94% of those surveyed nationwide know that walking is good for their health. They said it was a good way to lose weight, prevent heart disease, and also that walking reduced the incidence of anxiety and depression. However, 79% said they should walk more and 35% said that they were walking less than they did five years ago. However, almost a third of those surveyed said they walk more than they did five years ago. The U.S. Centers for Disease Control and Prevention recommends people walk at least 10 minutes a week.

It is essential that people give up their sedentary life styles if they want to have good health and physical fitness, and prevent many of the diseases that occur from the lack of exercise. It is a well-known fact that walking reduces the incidence of high blood pressure, heart disease, strokes, neurological diseases of aging and certain forms of cancer. Our bodies are made for walking, so come on people, no excuses, let's get out there and start walking like your life depended on it. It really does!

FEEL & LOOK YOUNGER

Walking produces a remarkable number of changes that occur inside of your body. Your blood volume and the red blood cells increase in number. Your *heart* pumps blood more efficiently. Your lungs expand, taking in and distributing more oxygen. Your muscles tighten and contract, giving you a firmer figure. Your energy level increases, and you feel strong and fit. The results of these changes will make your figure lean and your posture supreme. Your overall appearance will improve following your daily walk, since walking will improve your circulation and enable you to feel and look great. Your skin, complexion and hair texture will also improve with walking because of the increased blood circulation to the skin and hair follicles. Your complexion will literally glow after your walk and your skin will stay healthy and fresh looking all day long.

After you have been walking for a while you will notice that your muscles will become firm and many of the fatty deposits on your thighs and buttocks will start to decrease in size. Your stomach will become flatter and the muscles of your calves, thighs and buttocks will become firmer and shapelier. These changes result from improved muscle tone and also from the strengthening of muscles and ligaments, which are attached to the spine.

You don't have to kill yourself to stay fit, trim and healthy. Walking actually provides better long-term figure control and fitness benefits than jogging or other strenuous exercises, without the hazards and dangers. Always remember that exercise does not have to be painful or uncomfortable to be effective. The Philly Fit-Step Walking Diet consists of walking for 40 minutes, 6 days per week, and walking for 40 minutes using light, hand-held weights for 3 days per week provides the easy steps needed for a trim, beautiful body. Remember, two 20 minute walking sessions daily work just as well.

MOST OF US JUST SIT THERE!

Just think how many hours a day we waste in front of our TV sets. Or how many hours we sit at our desks and work every day. Consider the number of hours that we spend inside of our cars daily, going from here to there and everywhere. Do we ever go out for a walk? Do we spend any time moving our sedentary bodies? No, we just log on to the Internet, and spend hour after hour looking for anything and everything that in reality is "much ado about nothing." And no matter how you put it, all we do is "**just sit there**." Is it any wonder that we are an overweight, under-exercised society? Can there be any doubt that "just sitting there" is a major cause of a number of diseases, disability, and even premature death. We have been raised in the "just sitting there" mode, in part caused by the advances in technology, which leaves us very little to do that actually involves physical motion of any kind.

I know many of you at one time or another have joined a gym and made a real effort at exercise. But most of you have found that the time involved and the strenuous effort required only leads to frustration and ennui. After working all day, how can anyone keep up with the bionic, 20-year-old aerobics instructor? How can anyone continuously hop from machine to endless machine, so that each and every tiny muscle in our bodies is exercised to the maximum? Who in their right mind would attempt to lift weights that even Hercules would find difficult? And how can anyone after a long hard day at work, muster up the strength to run and run and even run faster on the mechanical motion monster machines that send our hearts pumping ever so fast, our blood pressure rising precipitously, and our muscles, ligaments and joints screaming "pain, pain, pain?" Is it any wonder why most of us finally give up our home exercise programs or our fitness club memberships, so that we can finally do what we have been genetically programmed to do all of our lives. "Let's just sit there. We really need our rest. I just don't have the time to exercise or work out. Those exercise machines were far too formidable and powerful for the likes of us. Yes, we concede the fact that the machines have won. Let's just sit there and rest."

Well let's not get too comfortable yet. We don't have to "just sit there." Even though the machines have beaten us, we can take heart in the fact that we are still alive, albeit maimed and weakened. And would you believe it, the machines don't even have as much as a scratch on them. But take heart my fellow exercisers; you actually have your own secret machine built into your mortal bodies. This machine will not harm or injure you. This machine will not break your bones and limbs. This machine will not elevate your blood pressure and heart rate to dangerous levels. This is your very own personal body machine that has been with you all of your lives, and very few of you know of its power and its benefits. Yes, this machine is made up of your blood and your heart and your ligaments and joints and your muscles and bones and the rest of your wonderful anatomy. **It's your very own friendly walking machine.** It's been there forever, and for whatever reason, it has been gathering dust in the cobwebs of your mind. You have never even considered what a powerful and awesome machine your walking machine can be.

To walk is what helps your life's blood circulate and provide oxygen to all of your body's cells. Walking aids in your digestion, in your metabolism, and in your breathing and circulation. Walking helps to lubricate and strengthen your muscles, joints and ligaments. Walking helps your heart to stay healthy, and walking supplies oxygen and nutrients to all of your body's cells. Walking keeps your brain supplied with oxygen so that you can finally realize what a powerful machine you had hidden away somewhere in the recesses of your brain, and walking is the secret code that can be used to overcome our genetic predisposition to "just sit there." By walking, we override the synapses in our brains that tell us that we should "just be sitting there." We actually now have the scientific technology to reprogram our "just-sitting-there genes," and in a sense alter our DNA. Now we will be able to get out of our chairs, out of our cars, out from in front of our computers and TVs, and propel us forward so that we can now move about freely without supervision or restriction. And then we can finally say, "Yes, I really can lose 15 pounds in 21 days, and become fit in spite of myself."

EASILY FIT BACK INTO YOUR JEANS

And as far as exercise is concerned, there is no doubt in anyone's mind that exercise is really a bore and most exercises usually are just too strenuous and time-consuming, Jump up, lift that, squat here, run there, or any one of a dozen useless body gyrations that leave us huffing and puffing. Or hop like a bunny on this machine or that one, so that you can exercise one tiny little muscle on each and every machine. You would essentially have to hop on a hundred different machines to exercise all of your muscle groups individually. Then you start thinking, "Did I exercise my triceps or was it my biceps?" "Was I already on that machine, or was that machine in a different row?" "To tell the truth, all of these machines look the same." "They're making me crazy; now I have to start all over again since I don't know where I began." "Maybe I should use free-weights, but what really are free weights?" All of this seems very confusing, and is easily remedied by just following the Philly Fit-Step Walking Diet.

Studies have repeatedly shown that strenuous exercises, rather than being beneficial, are actually detrimental to our health. Strenuous exercises and lifting heavy weights can actually raise our blood pressures and make us more susceptible to irregular heart rhythms. And of course, there is all of the muscle and joint and ligament injuries that all of these over enthusiastic exercisers sustain over and over again. Won't they ever learn? I think not. People have been brainwashed into thinking that if an exercise is not painful or strenuous, then it can't be good for you. This is the so-called "no-pain no-gain myth." Nothing could be further from the truth. Medical studies have repeatedly shown that moderate exercise is far more beneficial and less detrimental to our health than those back-breaking, gut-wrenching, limb-straining types of exercises.

You don't really have to join a gym or a fitness club to exercise. You don't have to engage in lung-straining, muscle-wrenching, heart-racing, anaerobic and aerobic exercises in order to lose weight and get fit. And you do not have to subject your body to all of the torturous exercises that the so-called fitness gurus have brainwashed everyone into believing are essential for weight loss and fitness. So what do we do? Just sit there! Not really! The answer is simple. You don't have to just sit there. All you have to do is follow **Philly's Fit-Step Walking Diet**, which consists of an easy-to-follow diet and exercise plan that will allow you **to lose up to 15 pounds and 3 inches and easily fit back into your jeans in just 21 days.**

POWER WALK INTO YOUR NEW FIGURE

Walking on **softer surfaces** like sand, dirt, or grass could help you burn an extra 100 calories in 40 minutes. This type of activity should be limited to one or two days per week.

Walk up hills as part as of your walking program on two or three days per week. This can help you burn an additional 150 calories in 40 minutes.

Walking on cobblestones or **uneven surfaces** uses different muscles than walking on a flat surface and burns more calories as you walk. It is important to be careful to walk carefully on these uneven surfaces to prevent ankle and/or foot strains or sprains. Also, be careful of unfortunate trips and falls.

Intermittent speed walking—Walk as fast as you can for two minutes and then slow down to your normal three miles per hour pace. Increase speed again after five minutes of your normal pace for another two minutes. Do this three or four times during your 40 minute walk, depending on your fatigue level. If you become fatigued or short of breath then just do your speed walking at one minute intervals. If fatigue, shortness of breath, chest pain, or any other symptoms occurs, discontinue speed walking and see your doctor immediately.

Be careful when increasing your walking speed, and resist the temptation to stretch your stride too far. If you stretch your stride too far, then you will throw off your balance while walking and put extra stress on your knees and shin bones.

Walk up and down **stairs** ten minutes every day in addition to your 35 minute walking program. This will burn an additional 100 calories per day.

Increase your **speed of walking** from 3.5 to 4 miles per hour for 10 minutes, and then resume walking at three miles per hour for the rest of your 40 minute walk. You can use a pedometer to calculate distance and speed of walking.

To **burn even more calories**, increase your speed from 3.5 per hour to 4.5 miles per hour for ten minutes, and then resume your walk at 3.5 miles per hour.

Stretch your stride so that your foot lands first on your heel and then on your sole all the way through your stride to end up on your toes. This stretching of your stride tones and firms leg muscles and burns additional calories.

Concentrate on **holding your tummy in** while you walk for several minutes, and then release your abdominal muscles. This burns additional calories and helps to melt belly fat.

There is no such thing as **"spot reduction"** while doing different exercises. For instance, you won't remove fat deposits in your buttocks on a stair climber or elliptical machine. Also, doing sit-ups won't remove excess fat around your waist. When you do a well-rounded exercise like walking or walking with light weights (Chapter 10), fat will be burned gradually from fat deposits all over your body

Increase your walking time from 40 minutes daily to anywhere between 45 to 90 minutes every day. This could burn significantly more calories each day. **Chapter 7-DIETWALK: Quick Weight-Loss Walking** shows you how to lose weight more quickly by increasing the time that you walk each day. You'll fit back into your jeans super-fast.

3 EASY STEPS TO WEIGHT-LOSS & FITNESS

The Philly Fit-Step Walking Diet is really an easy, safe and effective way to lose up to 15 pounds in 21 days. You will also become physically fit and shape your body as you follow this easy weight-loss and fitness plan. The basic essentials of the Philly Fit-Step Walking Diet are divided into three simple parts:

Step 1: The Diet-Step: 40/40 Plan simply consists of a **low-fat, high-fiber, moderate lean protein diet,** *with no more than 40 grams of fat and no less than 40 grams of fiber daily* And that's it! There are no special menus to follow, no complicated meals to prepare, and no restrictions on good tasting, nutritious healthy foods. The diet works equally well in a restaurant as it does at home. You will see from the meal plans that are included in the book that these plans can be easily changed to meet your own individual needs and tastes. You can mix and match any number of helpful, nutritious, good tasting foods for any of your meals. You will be delighted with all of the options you have, and none of the dietary restrictions that you have been made to follow on all of those gimmick diet plans floating out there in space and cyber space, which is where they actually belong and should stay. The Philly Fit-Step Walking Diet is really a fun diet and exercise plan, and one that you can easily and safely stay on for a lifetime. Just remember to eat at least 40 grams of fiber daily and limit your total fat intake to no more than 40 grams per day.

Step 2: The second part of the Philly Diet-Fit Walking Step is **The**

Fit-Step: 40 Minute Walking Plan. This step consists of an easy, moderate, **40 minute aerobic walking plan 6 days per week.** This walking plan can be done anytime, anywhere, or anyplace that you choose. In the morning, at lunchtime, after dinner, whenever it's convenient for you. It's your own plan. It is really quite simple. Walk at a brisk pace, approximately 3.5 miles per hour for 40 minutes, 6 days every week. Break it up into two 20 minute walks, if your time is limited. The choice is yours.

Step 3: Easy Strength-Training Exercises combines your 40 minute daily walking aerobic exercise with holding one pound hand-held weights as you walk every other day, 3 days per week. These weights come in several varieties. One type looks like brass knuckles turned inside out, where you grip the padded weights with the fingers of each hand in the indentations on the weights. The other variety of hand-held weights combines a strap that goes over the back of your hand, while you hold the weights in the palms of your hand. These weights look like mini-dumbbells. The combination of walking for 40 minutes using hand-held weights is only done three days per week. This should not be done on consecutive days because it puts too much strain on the upper body muscles.

This combination of walking using hand-held weights provides a double-blast of fat-burning calories. The reason for this is that you are burning calories by the aerobic action of walking, and you are also burning calories by the muscle-building action of the hand-held weights on your upper body. You are in a sense combining an aerobic exercise with a strength training exercise, all rolled up into one simple 40 minute walk. Sound easy? It is! And believe me; it works without any of the dangers or hazards involved in strenuous exercises or by using heavy weights for strength training and muscle building (Chapter 10).

How Your Body Burns Calories At Rest

A new study from Yale University has shown that exercise benefits your body even at rest. These researchers studied the oxygen used by the calf muscles of the legs of both athletes and sedentary people. This use of oxygen by the muscles is known as the oxidation rate, which shows how fast muscles are burning up the calories while you are at rest. The researchers found that the athletes burned up calories 54% faster than did sedentary people. However, they also found that both the athletes and the sedentary people produced the same amount of a chemical form of stored energy called ATP. This finding may help to explain why the athletes were able to stay trimmer and slimmer, since they burned additional calories while they were even at rest.

FAST EATERS GAIN WEIGHT FASTER

Researchers from Osaka University in Japan studied the eating habits and body mass of approximately 3500 men and women between the ages of 30 and 69. Those individuals who ate quickly, doubled their risk of being overweight. When you eat quickly, your appetite control mechanism in the brain does not have a chance to realize that you're actually full, and therefore you'll eat considerably more food until your hunger mechanism finally tells you that you're no longer hungry. Being overweight means that you are at higher risk for developing hypertension, heart disease, strokes, and even certain forms of cancer. This study emphasizes that if you are interested in losing weight, you should eat meals at a slower pace and stop eating before you feel completely full.

FLATTEN YOUR ABS WITH POWER BREATHING

A simple exercise to help tighten and flatten your abdominal muscles is to take a deep breath and tighten your abdominal muscles. Hold your muscles taut for approximately 3-5 seconds and then release the tension as your breathe out slowly. You can do this simple exercise while sitting at your desk, watching TV, or while you're driving your car. Begin with 5 abdominal tightening repetitions 3-4 times daily, and gradually build up slowly to 10-12 repetitions every other day over a 14 day period. Once you've reached 10-12 repetitions of abdominal tightening-deep breathing exercises after the first 2 weeks, then continue doing the abdominal flattening exercises every other day, in order to give your abdominal muscles time to rest between these abdominal tightening exercises. Remember, muscles need time to heal and regenerate, just like they do with any strength training, weight bearing exercises. You should space these 10-15 repetitions three to four times throughout the day. If you feel that it is too tiring, then decrease the number of repetitions until you feel comfortable.

SHAPE-UP WALKING

The following physical and physiological effects will be noted after you have been on your walking diet for 21 days. **Muscle tone** certainly is one of the most important results we are looking for. After your daily 40 minute walk, you will notice that your muscles will be toned and firm, and after you have been on your walking program for some time, you will notice many of the fatty bulges and deposits decreasing in size. Your stomach will flatten and your calves and thighs will become trimmer, and your buttocks muscles will become more proportioned. Many of these changes are due to improved muscle tone and, secondarily, to the strengthening of the spine.

- **Flatter stomach**—the abdominal muscles will be firm and support the intra-abdominal contents, so that the appearance will be of a flatter stomach.

- **Slender thighs**—leg strengthening and loss of fat in the thigh muscles will reduce the outer and inner thigh dimensions.

- **Firmer buttocks**—the large buttocks muscle, called the gluteus maximus, will contract and draw the buttocks higher and make them appear firmer.

- **Upper arms leaner and shapelier**—the muscles of the upper arm, which include the triceps and biceps, will increase their tone, and the fat loss from the fleshy part of the upper arm will combine to form a firmer, shapelier arm.

- **Firmer, higher appearing breasts**—the pectoral muscles of the chest will lift the breasts to make them appear larger, although they will not actually grow in size.

- **Increased level of energy**—with increased aerobic training, the lungs, heart, and circulation will be improved in efficiency and add more energy to your day.

- **Improved nightly sleep**—a regular walking program will aid in sleep without the use of sedatives or tranquilizers.

WALK AWAY STRESS

Regular exercise can help to abate the mental and physical effects that stress has on your body. Under stressful conditions, your body responds by producing stress hormones (**adrenaline** and **cortisol**), as well as releasing fatty acids and glucose, which are used as fuel to produce energy. This combination of stress hormones and fuel products are the body's response to stress, known as **"fight or flight phenomena."** Both short-term stress situations and long-term stress conditions, can lead to high blood pressure, coronary artery disease, and strokes. Also problems with digestion, headaches, anxiety, insomnia, depression, and a weakened immune system can result from long-term stress.

Physical exercise can aid the body to combat the effects of stress, by helping to burn up these stress hormones (adrenalin and cortisol) and by producing relaxing hormones called **endorphins**, which have a calming effect on the body's nervous system and help to elevate good mood feelings. Regular exercise, especially a moderate walking exercise program, helps the body combat the stress of everyday living. An aerobic exercise walking program makes you feel better and in turn helps you look better. Other relaxation activities, such as yoga and meditation, can also help you combat stress.

By combining a regular aerobic exercise walking program with strength-training exercises, using hand-held weights on the Philly Fit-Step Walking Diet, you will actually produce more endorphins, which will help your body dissipate the stress hormones. This combination is one of the best methods of dealing with stress and tension. As you continue on your Philly Fit-Step Walking Diet, your body will continue to burn calories and increase your metabolic rate. This increased metabolic rate will boost your energy level as it decreases your stress hormones and increases your relaxation hormones. Walk away stress and tension and let the feel-good hormones wash over your body.

STRENGTHEN BONES AND MUSCLES

Since the runner pounds the ground with a force equal to three to four times their body weight, she or he is more likely to sustain injuries than the walker. Walking is one of the most natural functions of the human body. Due to the structure of a person's musculoskeletal system and the shape and flexibility of the spine, the body is perfectly constructed for walking.

As you walk, the muscular and skeletal systems perform synchronously together. Your curved flexible spine has a spring-like function, made up of many vertebrae, each separated from the other by a tiny cushion (inter-vertebral disc), which is designed to absorb shock. These discs also give the spine its resilience and flexibility. When you walk, you use the hinge-like joints in your feet, ankles and knees while the ball and socket joints in your hips move effortlessly with a liquid-like motion.

The muscles that are attached to the long bones of the legs and the pelvis are specifically designed for walking. The leg, hip and back muscles are used for support and the mechanics of propelling the body forward. The long bones of the legs form a frame-work of levers, which are moved by these muscles, and subsequently help to propel the body forward. The abdominal muscles support the weight of the abdominal organs when you walk and your chest wall and diaphragm muscles assist in respiration.

As your legs thrust forward, you are in effect catching the forward motion of the upper part of your body. This natural motion in walking creates a perfect balance between gravity's force and the forward thrust of your body. The act of walking is therefore an almost effortless biodynamic mechanism, structurally more efficient than any woman or man-made machine. Just remember to swing your arms naturally when you walk. As you'll see in (Chapter 10), the combination of walking for 40 minutes, 6 days per week using hand-held weights for three days per week, will burn more calories, and will shape and strengthen your upper body muscles. The Philly Fit-Step Diet Strength-Training workout plan, is therefore the perfect body-shaping plan for muscle strengthening and toning, and quick weight-loss.

TRIM-STEP: BEACH TONING

It is possible to almost double the number of calories that you burn when you are walking on sand rather than on hard surfaces. The reason for this is that your feet sink below the surface of the sand and your muscles, ligaments and joints have to work harder to lift your feet out of the sand. During your 30 minute walk it is possible to burn an additional 100-150 calories by just walking on sand.

Muscle toning in the areas of the calves, thighs, buttocks, and abdomen is more efficient on sand. Again the reason for this is that the walking workout is more intense. Sand walking is great for beach toning which will enable you to look great in your bathing suit.

Wear a low cut walking sneaker to protect your feet from shells, rocks, glass and other beach debris. Keep your feet dry with light weight socks to protect against blisters; however, if you are brave enough, then walking barefoot can be a lot of fun if you are careful. Don't forget to use a good sun blocker to protect your skin from the sun's ultraviolet rays. Also be careful if you have any back, knee or ankle problems because of the excess strain put on these areas by the force transmitted by sand walking, which is a high intensity type of walking. Also the uneven walking surfaces that you encounter on sand sometimes can have an adverse effect on these problem areas. Stop if you develop pain in any area of the body, and begin again after you've rested. You may tire more easily because of the increased difficulty of walking in sand. If that is the case, stop and rest and then begin again.

PHILLY'S FIT-STEP WALKING DIET STRETCH

Stretching exercises can improve the flexibility of the joints, muscles and tendons, thus making the body less prone to injury. Stretching also increases the flow of blood to the stretched muscle and helps to promote bone growth where there is a stretching motion against gravity. There is increasing evidence that stretching has a calming effect on the central nervous system by transmitting relaxing signals along chemical neurotransmitter pathways from the peripheral nervous system to the brain.

Stretching should be done slowly, and stretching one muscle group at a time is preferable. For example, stretch both arms in front of you, and hold that position for 30 seconds and then let your arms down slowly, and relax them for an additional 30 seconds. Repeat this extension of both arms out to your sides, holding for 30 seconds, and then slowly letting them down and relaxing them for 30 seconds. Repeat this motion with your arms above your head, and then with your hands clasped in back of your head with your elbows bent, as if you are stretching when you get out of bed. During each of these exercises, gently stretch the arms, by actually pulling or pushing them away from the body, and then pulling them back towards the body. Remember to do it gently, and if it hurts, you're stretching your muscles too much.

Do the same procedure with your neck muscles. First look up and hold your head in that position for 30 seconds and then relax, returning to a normal head position for 30 seconds. Repeat the same procedure looking to the left, and then to the right. Repeat this looking down, with your chin resting on your chest for 30 seconds, and then return to the normal head position for 30 seconds. The best way to stretch your leg muscles and ligaments is to sit in a chair and stretch one leg at a time in front of you for 30 seconds, then relax the muscles, and then bend your knee, and hold that position for an additional 30 seconds, then relax the muscles and place your foot back on the floor. Repeat the same procedure with the other leg. You also can accomplish this by pressing your feet into a footrest while sitting on a plane, train, bus, or at your desk.

These simple stretching exercises are designed to develop maximum flexibility of the muscles, ligaments and joints. Although not as elaborate as yoga or tai-chi, they are effective limbering and toning exercises. These stretching steps help prepare the body for mental as well as physical fitness. They help you to get in touch with your body as you contemplate the slow, relaxing, stretching steps. Remember to take slow deep breaths during stretching exercises for maximum relaxing. You can develop any stretching routine that feels good to you, not just those described above. Stretching is an individual exercise, and what feels good for one person may not be satisfactory to another. You can also stretch by interlacing the fingers in front of your body, above your head or behind your back, while you do the simple stretching exercises described above.

Remember, if the stretching exercise hurts, either during or after the exercise, then you have stretched too vigorously. Go easy the next time. When you've finished, your muscles should feel relaxed, not taut or tight. The major advantage of the Philly Fit-Step Walking Diet Stretch is that it can be done any time, anywhere or any place. When you don't have the time to walk or the weather's inclement, stretching is a viable alternative to limbering up. Stretching can also be used to warm up your muscles before your 40-minute walk.

ACTIVE OLDER ADULTS

In a study reported in the *Journal of the American Medical Association,* researchers from the National Institute of Health reported that active older adults lived considerably longer than inactive older people. This study involving over 300 older adults measured the energy expended from normal daily activities such as housecleaning, climbing the stairs, gardening, shopping, baking, and working at home or outside the home and running around after the grandkids. These individuals who expended the most energy throughout the day had a 30% lower risk of dying during the six-year period than those people who expended less energy. As I have said over and over again, it does not matter whether you join a gym, take a walk, or just do your household chores, the results are the same. You do not have to run a marathon to become fit, all you have to do is incorporate energy-expending activities into your daily routine. This study found that those adults who were the most active were those who climbed at least two flights of stairs.

LIVE LONGER & LOOK YOUNGER

1. **Walking lowers blood pressure by:**

   A. dilating (opening) the arteries, allowing more blood to flow through

   B. improving elasticity of blood vessels, giving less resistance to the flow of blood

   C. lowering chemicals in blood that can raise blood pressure- (catecholamines and angiotensin)

D. improving return of blood to the heart, so that the heart can work more efficiently at a slower rate

E. increasing the amount of oxygen delivered to all tissues and cells

F. decreasing the rate of sodium reabsorption in the kidneys

2. Walking protects the heart by:

A. decreasing the risk of blood clot formation

B. Improving the return of blood to the heart from the leg veins

C. increasing the flow of blood through the coronary arteries

D. increasing HDL (good) cholesterol which protects the heart and arteries against fatty deposits (plaque)

E. improving the efficiency of the heart's cardiac output (total volume of blood pumped out by the heart each minute

F. helping to keep the collateral circulation open and available for emergencies.

3. Walking improves lung efficiency and breathing capacity by:

A. conditioning the muscles of respiration (chest wall and diaphragm)

B. opening more usable lung space (alveoli)

C improving efficiency of extracting oxygen from the air.

4. Walking improves the general circulation by:

A. increasing the total volume of blood, and the amount of red blood cells, allowing more oxygen to be carried in the bloodstream

B. dilating the arteries, thus improving blood flow

C. increasing flexibility of arteries, thus lowering blood pressure

D. compression of leg and abdominal veins by the pumping action of the muscles used in walking, aiding the return of blood to the heart

E. using small blood vessels in the legs for re-routing blood (collateral circulation) around blocked arteries in emergencies.

5. Walking prevents the build-up of fatty deposits (plaque) in arteries by:

A. decreasing the serum triglycerides (sugar fats)

B. decreasing LDL (bad) cholesterol in the blood

C. increasing HDL (good) cholesterol

D. preventing the blood from getting too thick, thus lessening the chance that blood clots

6. Walking promotes weight loss and weight control by:

A. directly burning calories

B. regulating the brain center (appestat) to control appetite

C. re-directing blood flow away from digestive tract toward the exercising muscles thus decreasing appetite

D. using blood fats instead of sugar as a source of energy

7. Walking controls stress by:

A. increasing relaxation hormones in the brain (Beta-endorphins) and decreasing stress hormones (epinephrine and norephrine).

B. increasing the oxygen supply and decreasing the amount of carbon dioxide to the brain

C. efficient utilization of blood sugar in the body regulated by an improved production of insulin

D. literally walking away from stress

8. Walking promotes a longer healthier life by:

A. strengthening the heart muscle and regulating the cardiac output (a slower more efficient heart rate)

B. lowering blood pressure, thus preventing strokes, heart attacks and kidney disorders

C. improving lungs' efficiency in extracting oxygen from air

D. improving the efficiency of the delivery of oxygen to all the body's organs, tissues and cells

E. strengthening muscle fibers throughout the body thus improving reaction time and maintaining muscle tone

F. maintaining bone strength and structure by preserving the mineral content of the bone, thus preventing osteoporosis (bone thinning).

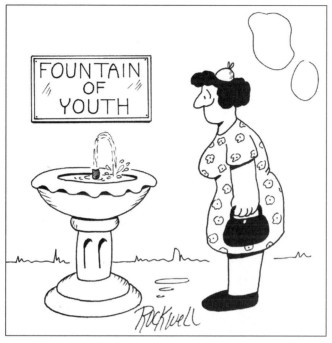

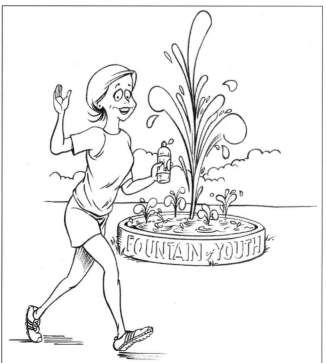

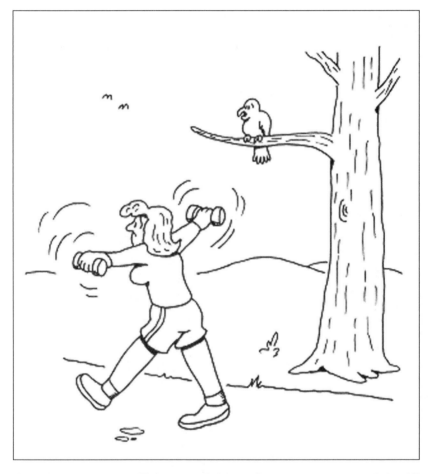

"You'll never get off the ground holding on to those weights!"

10

EASY BODY-SHAPING PLAN

BE FIT, FIRM & STRONG

Tell most people that walking produces a flat tummy, slim hips and thighs and they'll tell you that you're crazy. "You need to do strenuous calisthenics and exercises to reduce fat deposits in those areas." Don't' be too sure! When you also do the Fit-Step Walking Diet Workout Exercises using hand-held weights while walking, you'll quickly develop a trimmer more sculptured figure. First of all, when you walk briskly with an even stride you are contracting and relaxing muscles in your chest, back and abdomen. With each forward motion of your legs, these muscles contract to keep your body erect. Your abdominal muscles tighten automatically, exactly as they would if you were doing strenuous sit-ups, with one exception—you're not straining your back muscles. As you swing your upper arms, the upper chest wall muscles that are tied in with the upper abdominal wall muscles aid in tightening these abdominal muscles.

This combination of upper body and lower abdominal muscle contractions are what produce *a firm, flat tummy*. With repeated bouts of walking with hand-held weights come repeated bouts of muscle tightening, until a point is reached when your abdominal muscles are firm and taut all of the time, whether you're walking or not. This firm, flat tummy will continue to last as long as you walk regularly. Also as you walk, the forward and backward motion of each hip stretches the hip muscles. This hip motion tugs at your lower abdominal muscles, further flattening your tummy.

Now what about those lumpy, bumpy hips and thighs? First of all, don't let anyone give you the baloney about *"cellulite deposits."* There's no such thing as cellulite! It's a term coined by diet promoters to encourage people to purchase diet-gimmicks to rid themselves of the mythical cellulose. Microscopic studies of fat show that fat cells are connected by strands of connective tissue. When these connective tissue strands stretch, they lose their elasticity and subsequently the fat gives a lumpy appearance. Regular fat cells and the so-called cellulite fat deposits are indistinguishable under the microscope. *Fat is fat!* And cellulite is phony-baloney! Again, walking regularly combined with weight-resistance exercises will trim down those lumpy, bumpy hips and thighs.

Since walking is a moderate aerobic exercise, it burns fat rather than muscle tissue. The result: *trim hips and thin thighs.* When this walking fat-burning process is combined with weight-bearing exercises (hand-held weights), you will also lose those unsightly lumpy fat deposits. Sounds too easy? It certainly is! It's the **Philly Easy Body Shaping Plan.**

The forward motion of your legs results in the tightening of lower abdominal muscles also produces a tightening effect of your lower back and buttocks muscles. This combination of alternate muscle groups contracting and relaxing produces firm and tight buttocks muscles. This firming effect actually lifts the buttocks so that they lose their saggy appearance. Your thighs will also become firm and trim and will remain that way as long as you continue your 40 minute walking program 6 days per week and use your hand-held weights 3 days per week for strength-training.

Your posture will also improve as your shoulders and back muscles strengthen when you walk with hand-held weights. Your head will assume an erect position and your back and spine will straighten. Your buttocks and thigh muscles will tighten and firm up, and your upper arms will lose their flabby appearance. Your figure will slowly go through a metamorphosis and you will appear younger, feel better and be healthier than you ever were before.

However, it must be noted that these changes can only be sustained by continuing these exercises along with reducing the amount of dietary fat in your diet. And probably the best, most effective, and easiest way to develop tight abs, trim thighs, and firm buttocks, and strong upper body muscles, is to walk for 40 minutes, 6 days per week, and walk for 40 minutes using hand-held weights three days per week. You can also divide your walking into two 20 minute sessions.

STRENGTH-TRAINING BURNS FAT

Studies reported at the 2008 Experimental Biology Meeting, showed that short, simple, weight-training workouts helped men and women of all ages lose weight and keep that weight off permanently. Weight-training also was shown to strengthen the body's immune system, as well as lower the blood pressure. By following a low-fat, moderate protein and complex carbohydrate diet, combined with simple weight-training exercises for fourteen weeks, the participants in this study lost fat and weight, and increased the proportion of muscle to body weight. Also, these men and women showed significant improvement in blood pressure, heart rate, and aerobic fitness.

The basal metabolic rate like the energizer bunny keeps on ticking even after you have stopped walking. Your body's normal resting basal metabolic rate burns approximately one calorie per minute (CPM). During your regular 40 minute daily walk at 3.5 miles per hour, your basal metabolic rate increases to five calories per minute. When you stop walking your basal metabolic rate does not return to its resting one calorie per minute rate. Your body's metabolic rate got so revved up from your 40 minute walk it continues to remain elevated for up to six hours after you have stopped walking. This increased rate will not remain at five calories per minute, but it will stay at between two to three calories per minute for the next six hours. What does all that mean? Well, if you walk for one half hour during lunch, when you get back to the office and are stuck behind your computer for the rest of the day, your body's metabolic rate will be burning two to three calories per minute instead of burning the usual sedentary one calorie per minute. The same process will occur if you take a one half hour walk after supper. You will actually be burning an additional two to three calories per minute while you are sleeping rather than the resting one calorie per minute metabolic rate. This actually means that you will burn more calories every day while you walk and also at rest after you walk. In effect, you have discovered a *double blast of calorie burning*. You burn calories with exercise and then you continue to burn calories when you stop exercising. Your body is actually giving you a bonus for exercising.

IMPORTANCE OF STRENGTH-TRAINING

A new study by the American Heart Association recommends resistance training for people with or without cardiovascular disease. It shows there are considerable benefits to improving muscular strength beyond the benefits of a regular aerobic exercise walking plan. Lifting weights or exerting force against resistance is an integral part of an overall exercise program for weight reduction and cardiovascular fitness.

Both resistance training and aerobic exercise (walking) have different positive effects on fitness development in your body. For example:

- Aerobic exercise (walking) has a moderate effect on the percentage of body fat, and a major effect on cardiovascular fitness.

- Resistance training has a moderate effect on lean body mass and major affects on muscular strength, while aerobic exercise has little effect on both.

- Both aerobic exercise and resistance training produce similar beneficial effects on both the HDL and the LDL cholesterol, whereas aerobic exercise has a greater effect on lowering serum triglycerides.

Resistance training is now fairly well recognized in cardiac rehabilitation programs. People with a history of heart failure or heart disease can improve their functional capacity, physical strength, endurance, and the quality of their lives, by the addition of strength training exercises to their aerobic walking exercise program. This type of exercise, which includes strength-training exercises, especially in the elderly, must be under careful medical supervision.

You're Never Too Old To Strength Train

According to the American Heart Association, strength training exercises can even help nursing home residents gain strength for everyday living. In a 10 week resistance training program, elderly nursing home residents, even those with a previous history of heart attacks or heart failure, have been shown to be able to increase their strength by 43%, and their distance walked in 6 minutes by 49%. These resistance training exercises included abdominal crunches, lifting light weight dumbbells, and using hand-held weights while walking. This study recommended that elderly people begin with low levels of strength training and gradually increase the number of repetitions before adding additional weight or resistance.

This particular study, which was reported in a recent issue of the *Journal of Circulation*, stated that resistance training, whether it was doing sit-ups or lifting weights, should be used as a complement to a regular aerobic exercise program for maximum cardiovascular benefits. It is important to note, that these elderly patients must be under careful medical supervision, before, during and after performing strength-training exercises.

Build Muscle Mass

Men and women after 35 to 40 years of age begin to lose muscle mass at a rate of approximately one-third pound per year. Strength training exercises makes your muscles stronger and strengthens your bones. The muscle and ligaments attached to your bones create a traction or tension on the bones when you exercise. This traction causes your bones to strengthen, by helping to absorb more calcium into the bones from the bloodstream. This process increases the mineral content of the bones, thus strengthening your bones and making them less brittle.

Aerobic exercise is great for cardiovascular fitness and burning calories, but it does not build body muscle mass. Unless we exercise, fat replaces muscle as we age. The necessity for strength training is even more pronounced in women because they begin with more fat cells and less muscle tissue compared with men. Strength training is therefore essential for weight control, strong bones and muscles and overall fitness and well-being in everyone over the age of 35 to 40 years.

Many studies have shown that people who engage in strength training exercises develop an increase in skeletal muscle mass, whereas sedentary people lose considerable muscle mass over a period of time. Bone mineral density also increases by 1.5% with strength-training and decreases by 2.5% in sedentary people. Also, these studies showed that strength-training in both men women increased their lean muscle mass by 4% and decreased their fat mass by 8%. This means that your muscles will become more shapely and defined and you will feel stronger because your muscles are actually stronger. You will have greater joint flexibility and have more energy when you walk. Your bones will be structurally stronger and, you will be less likely to develop osteoporosis or thinning of the bones as you get older.

Weight resistant exercises build your body's muscle mass. Improved muscle mass burns more calories by boosting your metabolism. When you build up your lean muscle mass, you can actually burn 35% more calories with exercise then you can if you were not doing strength training or strength resistance exercises. *Muscle cells are more efficient at burning calories than fat cells.*

On the other hand, if you just diet without exercising, you can actually lose muscle mass and subsequently decrease your basal metabolic rate. This means in effect that your basal metabolic rate slows down, so that even if you reduce your calorie intake, you will probably lose very little, if no weight at all. If you just add walking, you will increase your basal metabolic rate to five calories per minute, and if you add strength training exercises, you will increase your basal metabolic rate to six to seven calories per minute as you build muscle mass. This is the main reason that most people who do not exercise cannot lose weight, or if they do lose weight initially, they plateau and the weight remains the same. Only by using the combination of an aerobic exercise like walking and an anaerobic exercise like strength training with hand-held weights can you actually lose weight effectively and permanently. And only then can you break through the so-called impossible plateau that happens with each and every diet.

PHILLY'S SECRET MUSCLE BUILDER

You may think that the only way to build muscle mass is to do strength or weight training exercises. Or you may think that it's necessary to consume more protein in your diet in order to build muscle mass. You're correct on both counts; however, there's another secret sure-fire way to help build muscle mass, which is to consume *potassium rich foods* such as bananas, cantaloupes, sweet potatoes, pumpkin, avocado, oranges, tomatoes, sweet potatoes, winter squash and apricots. All of these fruits and vegetables can be found in Philly's Italian Market or at the famous Philadelphia Reading Terminal Market, or at any market in any city or town where you live.

Potassium appears to counter the effects of certain foods such as meats and refined grain cereals and breads, which create acid residues in the body that leads to muscle wasting. These fruits and vegetables, on the other hand, become alkaline in the body when digested, which in effect, neutralizes the acidity of other foods.

As we age, our muscle mass declines slowly after the age of 45. However, in a recent study, people over the age of 50 who ate lots of potassium rich foods gained approximately 2.5 more pounds of lean tissue muscle mass than those who consumed one half as much potassium.

DOUBLE BLAST OF CALORIE BURNING

Weight resistance exercises can include weight lifting, sit-ups, push-ups, aerobic exercises, swimming with flippers, or walking with hand-held weights. Of all the weight resistant exercises, walking with hand-held weights is the most efficient and safest weight resistance exercise. That is because it combines the aerobic fitness benefits of walking with the strength training exercises of hand-held weights. You actually have a double blast of calorie burning by walking with hand-held weights. First you burn calories by the aerobic exercise of walking, and secondly, you burn additional calories by building muscles using strength training exercises. It is also the easiest type of weight training since you are not subjecting yourself to strenuous exercises or heavy weights, which can make you prone to injuries.

In addition to this double blast of calorie burning and energy boosting exercise, you get a double reward from your body. As we previously said, when you stop walking your basal metabolic rate does not decrease to the resting one calorie per minute rate. The basal metabolic rate stays at about two to three calories per minute for up to six hours after you stop walking. But now that you have added weight resistance in the form of hand-held weights to walking program, you are actually building additional muscle mass. And as we said previously, muscle burns calories at a faster rate than fat cells and therefore you will burn additional calories after you have stopped using the hand-held weights. This means at rest, you can add another one calorie per minute burn to your walking with weights program. This translates into approximately three to four calories per minute burned when you are at rest after you have walked with hand-held weights. Have you ever noticed how fit, trim, muscular toned individuals can eat considerably more than unfit individuals. The reason for this is that they are always burning calories either during exercise or at rest.

WALKING WITH WEIGHTS

I usually recommend 1-pound cushioned hand-held weights, with either straps attached that go around the back of your hands, or hand-held weights with grooves for your fingers to grip the weights. If you're looking for more muscle definition and body-shaping, then after 4-6 weeks you can increase the hand-held weights to 2-pound weights. If you find that two pound hand-held weights are too heavy, then just continue your walking with weights program using one pound weights. These weights should be cushioned and covered with rubber or vinyl, since they won't rust and aren't cold to grip in cold weather. You can also purchase comfortable held-weights that are cushioned weights with soft-foam grips and secure hand straps.

A sure fire way to boost your calorie burning workout is to walk with hand-held weights. Using hand-held weights makes you work harder and improves your cardiovascular conditioning while building your upper body strength. Always check with your doctor before walking with hand-held weights, especially if you have any medical condition. Also be especially careful if you have back or joint problems before walking with hand-held weights and if you find it causes any pain or discomfort, then discontinue using weights while walking.

When you start your walking with weights program, take 10 minute walks every other day for the first 7 days, so that you don't over stretch your muscles and joints. Then build up to 20 minute walking with weights every other day for the next 7 days. After that, walk for 30 minutes every other day for the next 7 days. Starting at day 21, you can start your 40 minute walk with hand-held weights, three times a week. Initially, avoid any hills during your first six weeks while walking with hand-held weights to avoid over stressing or over stretching your muscles and joints.

Walk with a normal arm motion as you would walk without weights. Swing your arms close to your body in a short arc. Be careful not to over swing your arms as you can increase the risk of tendon, ligament and muscle injuries if the weights are swung in an exaggerated arc, especially above the shoulder areas. It is important to develop a walking stride and arm swing that is comfortable for you. Do not swing your arms faster than you would if you were walking naturally without weights. Also do not swing your arms at a slower rate than you would swing than without weights because they will create a dead load on your ligaments and joints and make them prone to injury.

Walking three times a week is all that is necessary to build upper body strength and muscle mass. Even after you walk with weights you will continue to burn calories at a faster rate than you would if you had just walked without weights. This is because your metabolism continues to burn excessive calories even after you are finished with your exercise. Walkers burn approximately 25% more calories doing the Philly Fit-Step Walking Diet using hand-held weights. Also, walking with weights *builds lean muscle mass, which burns an additional 50 calories an hour per 1 pound of muscle.* This activity is excellent for people of all ages and helps to maintain strong rotator cuff and shoulder muscles. Walking with weights also helps to develop good muscle tone, which improves balance and stability when walking. Also, walking with hand-held weight helps you to develop good posture and strong chest and abdominal wall muscles.

The **Easy Strength-Training Exercises** are the ideal combination of an aerobic exercise, which also adds upper body strength training. There is no need to engage in strenuous aerobic exercises or to lift heavy weights at the gym (either free weights or machine weights) in order to achieve cardiovascular fitness, weight loss, and improved lean muscle mass. Your body will burn fat as you lose weight and you will develop a new and improved, lean and firm figure. This results from the aerobic fat-burning exercise of walking, and the muscle-building exercise of walking with weights. For people who have reached a plateau in weight loss, the ideal fat burner is walking with hand-held weights

These changes occur because of the combination of the fat-burning aerobic walking exercise and the strength-training, upper body muscle-building exercise, when you use hand-held weights while walking. This is a combination that is truly impossible to reproduce. You don't have to do separate aerobic and strength-training exercises at different times or on different days. It's all combined in one easy, user-friendly exercise. These exercises are ideal in helping to prevent osteoporosis, since walking with hand-held weights puts the necessary tension on the bones and muscles, which is essential in preventing bone loss. Philly's Fit-Step Walking Diet Strength-Training plan of walking with weights is essential in helping to lose weight, improve cardiovascular fitness, lower blood pressure and also helping to reduce the incidence of heart disease and strokes.

Always check with your own physician to see if he/she feels that you are physically healthy and fit to walk with hand-held weights.

STRENGTH-TRAINING

Weight resistance exercises are good for your muscles and especially good for the body's most important muscle—your heart. In a recent study by the American Heart Association, it was reported that strength training exercises can significantly lower blood pressure. Those individuals who regularly lifted light weights experienced a reduction in the systolic blood pressure (when your heart muscles contract) and a reduction in the diastolic blood pressure (when your heart muscles relax). Their resting blood pressures dropped regardless of a person's body size or weight, or whether they used heavy weight resistance exercises with longer rest periods or lighter weight exercises with shorter rest periods. In other words, using lighter weights as we suggest in the **Philly Fit-Step Walking Diet,** causes the same reduction in blood pressure as those people who are lifting heavier weights. And actually lifting heavy weights can be dangerous to your health, because over the long run they can actually raise your blood pressure. Weight resistance exercises particularly using lighter weights as in the Fit -Step Strength-Training Plan is safe and effective, for weight reduction and building strong bones and muscles.

The American Heart Association's finding in their latest study showed that weight resistance exercises should be of moderate intensity. In other words instead of the fallacy "no pain-no gain," the truth as I've always told my patients, is "train, don't strain." Walking with weights makes your body leaner and your muscles more defined and sculptured. In addition, this plan builds stronger bones and muscles, straightens your posture, and strengthens your joints and ligaments. This plan also boosts your metabolism, which in turn helps you to lose weight. And finally, strength-training exercises enhance your sense of well-being and your self-confidence. So you will see that these strength-training exercises not only make you feel and look great, but help to strengthen your heart and lower your blood pressure.

FIT-STEP® BODY-SHAPING TIPS

1. WALKING WORKOUT

No matter how long you walk, your upper body, particularly your arms, shoulders chest and upper abdomen, get a free ride. Walking is not enough to build upper body strength. Even if you pump your arms vigorously while you walk, your upper body does not get stronger because there is no resistance to encounter while you walk. On the Fit-Step Plan however, your legs get stronger because they encounter the resistance of the ground and thus support your body's weight. In other words your legs get stronger, your thighs, buttocks and hips get firmer and your abdomen gets flatter on the Fit-Step Walking Diet.

Adding weight resistance using hand-held weights while walking is a great way to put your arms to work and to strengthen your upper body muscles. This combination of walking with hand-held weights actually makes you a stronger walker. A walker's upper body should be geared towards strength and endurance, not building muscle bulk. In other words, we want to sculpt and mold the upper body (arms, back and chest). Therefore, the key to the Fit-Step Walking Diet workout plan is to use light-weight, hand-held weights while walking 3 days per week, while you continue your 40 minute walking plan for 6 days every week. Divide this into two 20 minutes sessions daily if that's more convenient or you. This plan provides the unique power combination of strength training and aerobic fitness conditioning.

2. WILL WEIGHT TRAINING MAKE YOUR MUSCLES BULK-UP?

Many women have the misconception that weight training will result in building ugly massive muscles. Nothing could be further from the truth. In reality, women don't have to fear developing bulky muscles because of the increase in basal metabolic rate which occurs during the Philly Fit-Step Walking Diet. Strength training exercises actually burn more calories than fat and your muscles become more defined, as your muscle tissue replaces fat cells. Since women have more body fat than men, they are less likely to bulk up like men who have more muscle mass to begin with. Women will see improvement in muscle tone and strength after only 21 days on the Philly Fit-Step Walking Diet strength training exercises. Muscles will become more defined and sculptured for a trim, firm look in both men and women.

3. How the Fit-Step Diet Helps You Lose Weight.

As you walk with light-weight, hand-held weights you build muscle mass, which in turn speeds up your metabolism. Your muscle tissue burns more calories than fat cells burn; therefore, building muscle helps to boost your resting metabolism. This increase in the resting metabolism occurs because of the actual increased muscle mass that you develop and the increased metabolic activity in the muscles themselves. By combining your 40 minutes of aerobic walking with strength-training exercises using hand-held weights, you have the advantage of a "power blast" of calorie burning for weight loss, while you're actually firming and toning your body's muscle mass.. First of all, the aerobic walking at 3.5 mph in the Fit-Step® plan burns approximately 350 calories per hour or 235 calories every 40 minutes. The strength training exercises in the Philly Fit-Step Walking Diet plan burn an additional 200 calories per hour or approximately 100 extra calories every 30 minutes, which is accomplished just by increasing the body's basal metabolism. So you see you can actually lose more weight, more quickly by walking with hand-held weights.

4. Who Benefits from Walking with Weights?

Studies reported at the 2008 Experimental Biology Meeting, showed that simple weight-training workouts helped *men and women of all ages* lose weight and keep that weight off permanently. Weight-training also was shown to strengthen the body's immune system, as well as lower the blood pressure. By following a low-fat, moderate protein and complex carbohydrate diet, combined with simple weight-training exercises for fourteen weeks, the participants in this study lost fat and weight, and increased the proportion of muscle to body weight. Also, these men and women showed significant improvements in blood pressure, heart rate, and aerobic fitness.

Another similar study showed that middle-aged and elderly people developed stronger muscles and a healthier immune system while walking regularly, combined with light weight-training exercises. Many of the middle-aged and elderly people in this study were moderately obese when they started the program. After twelve weeks, the majority of the obese participants had lost considerable weight, in addition to gaining lean muscle mass. These individuals also developed improved cardiovascular fitness, in addition to gaining muscle strength and boosting their energy levels.

5. WHO SHOULD NOT WALK WITH WEIGHTS?

Individuals with has a medical condition such as coronary artery disease, heart disease, severe hypertension, cerebral or vascular disease and any other medical condition that their physician feels would be contraindicated by walking with weights. Also, people who have a neurological disorder, a degenerative or neuromuscular disease, or severe arthritis in any joint or in the spine should not walk with weights. In general, anyone who participates in the Philly Fit-Step Walking Diet Plan, with or without walking with weights, should first have a complete medical examination from their physician.

6. IMPROVE STRENGTH AND MUSCLE TONE

The Fit-Step Walking Diet strength-training plan is actually a walking aerobic exercise combined with an upper body strength-training exercise. As you walk with hand-held weights, you will burn an additional 25% more calories than you would burn by just walking. Walking with hand-held weights also builds lean muscle mass, which in itself burns an additional 50 calories per hour for every one pound of muscle. Walking with weights also helps to develop good muscle tone, which helps to improve balance and stability as you walk. And lastly, walking with weights also helps to develop strong arm, shoulder, chest and upper abdominal wall muscles, which in turn significantly improves your posture.

7. Boost Energy and Improve Fitness

The Fit-Step Diet strength-training is the ideal combination of an aerobic walking exercise combined with strength training using hand-held weights. It is not necessary to go to the gym in order to lift heavy weights (free weights or machine operated weights) or to engage in strenuous aerobic exercises. Just by simply walking with hand-held weights 3 days per week for 40 minutes, or two 20 minute sessions, you can achieve maximum cardiovascular fitness, burn calories, lose weight, and improve your lean body muscle mass. You will increase your metabolic rate as you burn fat, lose weight and boost your energy level. This combination of the aerobic fat-burning exercise of walking and the strength-training exercise of hand–held weights, is what causes you to lose weight quickly, develop a lean firm figure and develop strong bones and muscles. This plan will also help to improve cardiovascular fitness, lower blood pressure and reduce the incidence of heart disease and strokes.

PHILLY'S FIT-STEP® WALKING WORKOUT

1. Natural Arm Swing

This is the most common arm motion that you will use naturally when walking. When you just walk without weights your arms fall into a natural, not forced, swing at the side of your body. When you walk with hand-held-weights, your arms should also hang down at your side close to your body, holding the weights with your palms facing your body. As you walk, alternately swing your arms gently, as you bend your elbows ever so slightly. This is the natural arm swing motion of walking that you will be using all of the time during your regular 6 day per week, 40 minute Fit-Step® walking plan. This is a natural arm swing that is a motion that is most comfortable for you. Using the hand-held weights with this simple arm swing motion strengthens your triceps and upper shoulder muscles.

2. Locomotive Arm Motion

This is the arm motion that you see runners or fast walkers use while they are running or walking fast. Hold your arms close to your body and bend your arms at approximately a 90 degrees angle at the elbow, so the that your hands are making a slight fist facing in front of you. Hold the weights with palms facing your body. Now, do the locomotive! Start to move your arms alternately forward and backward. This motion strengthens the muscles of your upper arm, triceps and shoulder muscles.

Just do this exercise for a few minutes at a time during your 40 minute walk, and then go back to the natural arm swing. You can increase the number of minutes that you do the Locomotive Arm Motion as you develop more upper body strength, after you've been walking with weights for many weeks. Do not continue with this exercise if it initially causes muscle strain or pain. If you just work into it very gently, you will be able to build upper body strength gradually on the Philly Fit-Step Walking Diet.

3. HAMMER CURL SWING

This exercise begins exactly like the first natural arm swing exercise. Keep your arms hanging down at your sides close to your body, holding the weights with your palms facing your body. As you walk, bend each arm alternately at the elbow, towards your shoulder, and then lower each arm to the side of your body. Be sure to keep your arms close to your body. Pretend you're hammering a nail into a piece of wood or banging your fists on to a table top. This exercise strengthens your forearm and biceps muscles.

It is important to only do this exercise for a few minutes at a time during your 40 minute walk, and gradually build up the number of minutes using the Hammer Curl as you slowly improve your upper body strength over a period of many weeks on the Philly Fit-Step Walking Diet. Remember to revert to the Natural Arm Swing motion when you stop the Hammer Curl. Also, discontinue this exercise if it causes any pain or strain on your muscles and try it again at a later date.

This exercise is much safer to do while walking than is the traditional biceps curl, where your palms face away from your body and your wrists are rotated outward. You will prevent the hand-held weights from bumping your legs as you walk when you do the hammer curl instead of the traditional biceps curl. Also, you get better muscle strengthening and toning with this exercise.

FIT-STEP WALKING DIET WORKOUT EXERCISE TIPS

- **Start with 1-pound weights** in each hand three times per week for the first 21 days, and then you can build up to 2-pound weights if you really want more muscle definition and body shaping. If you find however, that 2-pound weights are too heavy or you tire easily, just stay with the 1-pound weights. Studies show that you still will get the same great muscle strengthening, toning and sculpting with very light weights. Actually most people do just fine with one pound weights.

- **Tighten your abdominal muscles** intermittently while you're doing these exercises while walking. This helps to provide support for your upper body and back, while helping to trim, tone and flatten your abdominal muscles.

- **How would you like to lighten your load** as you continue on your Fit-Step 40 minute walk? Instead of using hand-held weights, you can occasionally carry one 20 ounce plastic bottle of water in each hand. As you proceed on your 40-minute walk, you can drink from each bottle alternately, until each bottle becomes lighter and lighter. When you're finished with your workout, you will be refreshed and rehydrated. If you decide to take two 20 minute walks instead, then carry one 12 ounce plastic bottle of water in each hand.

- **How Many Repetitions Should You Do With Each Exercise?** You'll be able to customize the number of repetitions for each exercise depending on your own comfort level. During the first 21 days on the Philly Fit-Step Walking Diet, it's only necessary to do one set of 10-12 repetitions for each exercise. This is usually adequate strength training, as you rotate from one exercise to another. Then you should revert to your Natural Arm Swing motion of walking for the rest of your 40-minute or two 20 minute walks. Remember to start slowly with fewer repetitions when you start your walking workout and gradually build up the number of repetitions until you reach your own comfort level. You can gradually increase or decrease the number of repetitions after the first 3 weeks depending on your level of comfort.

If you find that either the locomotive arm motion or the hammer curl swing cause your arms or shoulders to become sore, then discontinue them and switch back to the normal arm swing. Walking with weights has to be done gradually in order to build up muscle strength without causing discomfort.

- **How Often Should You Walk With Weights?**
Many studies in exercise physiology show that strength training exercises two or three days per week, will prevent damage to muscle fibers that need time to heal after being stressed with weight resistance exercises. Also, by varying the strength-training exercises to different muscle groups, it helps to provide exercise to all of the upper body's muscles on a graduated basis. The significance of the Power Diet-Step® Strength Training exercises is that they are done while you are walking using very light weights. This considerably decreases the likelihood of muscle and ligament injury and eliminates the need to go to the gym for time-consuming, back-breaking, weight lifting routines. The latest research in exercise physiology has definitely shown that working-out different muscle groups only two or three times a week offers the same strength and muscle-firming benefits, as working out these muscle groups three or four times per week.

Therefore, on your regular Fit-Step Walking Diet plan, you will be walking for 40 minutes, six days per week. In the beginning, it will only then be necessary to use hand-held weights on two days each week on your walking workout. As you continue your Fit-Step walking with weights program, you can increase the number of days to three days per week after the first 21 days. Your walking workout with hand-held weights, three times per week will then result in more muscle toning, sculpting and strengthening. However, if you feel three times per week is too tiring or your muscles become sore, then walk with the weights only two times a week and just use the one pound weights instead.

- **The Easy Body-Shaping Workout**
  This workout does not involve lifting heavy free weights or working with complicated weight-machines at the gym. This easy plan features a unique combination of 40-minutes or two 20 minutes of aerobic exercise-walking six days per week, combined with walking two or three days per week using hand-held weights for strength-training. These light weights strengthen and build upper body muscles and bones as you walk, while burning additional calories by boosting your body's metabolism. This combination of an aerobic exercise and strength training delivers a double-blast of calorie burning, for complete cardiovascular fitness, maximum weight-loss and complete body-shaping.

- Make sure that you get a **complete physical examination** from your own physician before starting any phase of the Philly Fit-Step Walking Diet, especially the strength-training exercises.

WHAT'S THE BEST TIME TO DO THE FIT-STEP WORKOUT?

You can do your walking aerobic workout exercise any time of the day that's convenient for you. It's your schedule, so make it any time that you'd like. You can also change the times that you exercise each day depending on your own individual work schedule or home activities. Here are the pros and cons of exercising at various times of the day according to the so-called fitness experts. Take it with a grain of salt and individualize your own schedule to your own liking.

Morning —The main obstacle in the morning is getting out of bed. Once you're up, depending on if you're an early riser or not, you may want to leave yourself enough time so that you won't be rushed, especially if you have to go to work or have home responsibilities.

Since there are usually few disruptions in the A.M., women and men who walk in the morning are more likely to stick with their exercise plans over a long period of time. Plus, the sense of accomplishment, having completed your exercise early in the day, gives you a psychological rush for the first part of the day.

Afternoon —Many people feel an energy lag between two and three P.M. in the afternoon, which is related to the body's natural circadian rhythm. It may also be partly due to having just eaten lunch. Some exercise physiologists say that walking mid-day can smooth out that energy lag by increasing the levels of certain hormones that will perk you up for several hours. Remember, however, that it is not a good idea to exercise immediately after lunch or to skip lunch altogether. Walking for 30 minutes and then eating a light lunch will boost your energy level for the rest of the day.

Evening —Due to fluctuations in biological rhythms, it is in the late afternoon or early evening when your breathing is easier because your lungs' airways open wider, your muscle strength increases due to a slightly higher body temperature, and your joints and muscles are at their most flexible. This may also be a good time to walk according to some exercise physiologists. However, if you've had an extremely difficult day, and if you're dead tired, then revving yourself up for exercise may seem more like a chore than fun. Also, never exercise near bedtime, since the increased energy levels that follow the exercise may make it difficult to fall asleep. Determine the best time to do your workout according to your own biological clock and how you feel, and also according to your own time schedule. It's your body, so listen to it, and it will respond to you with boundless energy when you do the Philly Fit-Step Walking Diet.

CARDIO AND STRENGTH TRAINING COMBO

When you combine a cardiovascular workout with strength training exercises into one exercise routine, you save time, which is a great factor for most people whose time is limited.

Secondly, this cardio and strength training combo boosts the cardiovascular benefits and increases the aerobic calorie burning from walking, while doing upper body exercises. This double-blast of cal-orie-burning increases the amount of weight that you can lose in one half the time, not to mention the added health benefits of improved cardiovascular fitness.

Walking with light-weight, hand-held weights is the perfect ef-fective combination for cardiovascular and strength training. Unfortunately, there are some people who have tried to vary this car-dio strength training exercise using elastic arm bands wrapped around the console of a treadmill or an elliptical machine. This strenuous combination can increase your heartbeat and breathing too rapidly and puts excessive stress on your cardiovascular system. These elas-tic bands could also affect your normal gait on a treadmill, and will cause you to burn fewer calories because this activity will make you slow down. In addition, this awkward exercise combination can cause added stress and strain in your upper body's ligaments and tendons, and make you more prone to stress injuries.

Also, most elliptical machines, stationary bikes, and treadmills with arm levers that pull back and push forward, do very little to de-velop upper body strength. They only provide passive motion for your upper arms and can actually interfere with your normal gait and cause shoulder and upper body and arm injuries.

Once You're Fit, it Takes Longer to Get Out of Shape

"What if I can't keep up with the exercise plan regularly?" "What if I have to stop for a few days or a week or even longer if some inter-ruption in my life prevents me from continuing?" This is the kind of thinking that prevents many men and women from starting an exer-cise program and prevents others from going back to one that they've already begun. Never fear, the answer's here —**"It takes much lon-ger to get out of shape than it does to get into shape."**

The Philly Fit-Step Walking Diet is forgiving. Even if you miss a few days or a week or a few weeks in a month, there is no need to worry. Once you have been conditioned physically, it takes a lot longer to get out of shape than it took you to get into shape. The rate of regression depends on how long you've been exercising and how fit you are. The body is remarkable, since it tends to hold on to these fitness gains long after you've stopped exercising. Most women and men lose muscle strength at about one-half the rate at which they gained it. So, if you've been doing your aerobic walking program and your strength-training exercises for three months, and have to discontinue for any reason, it could take up to six months for your body to fall back to its pre-training state.

Aerobic capacity starts to decrease in the first two to three weeks after you've stopped exercising, but it can take up to six to eight months before fit exercisers get back to the fitness level where they started. Aerobic exercising (walking) decreases the LDL (bad cholesterol) and increases the HDL (good cholesterol) after you've been on your walking program for approximately two to three months. Studies show that it took at least three months for these cholesterol levels to return to their original pre-walking workout levels after the walking was discontinued.

That's pretty good, considering you've stopped walking all that time. When walkers resume their walking program, it took them only one-half the time to return to their original levels of fitness. So, don't worry if you have to discontinue your walking program for any reason or for any period of time. The benefits that you've worked so hard for are long lasting and they are easily obtained again in one half the time. *The Philly Fit-Step Walking Diet is forgiving and it keeps on giving!*

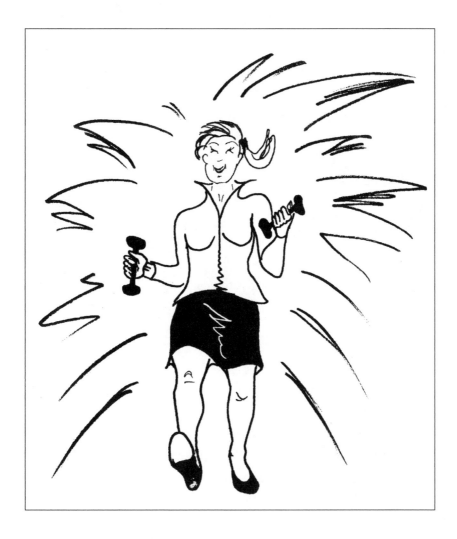

BIBLIOGRAPHY

Aburto, N.J. et al. "Effect of Increased Potassium Intake on Cardiovascular Risk Factors and Disease: Systematic Review and Meta-Analysis." *BMJ.* 2013 April 4; 346: fl378

Aburto, N.J. et al. "Effect of Lower Sodium Intake on Health: Systematic Review and Meta-Analysis." *BMJ.* 2013 April 4; 346; f126.

Artaud, F. et al. "Unhealthy Behaviors and Disability in Older Adults: Three-City Dijon Cohort Study. *BMJ.* 2013 July 23; 347: f4240.

Block J.P. et al. "Consumers' Estimation of Calorie Content at Fast Food Restaurants: Cross Sectional Observational Study." *BMJ* 2013 May 23; 346: f2907.

Azimi, A. et al. "Obesity Paradox Seen with CAD." *Family Practice News* 2013 October 15; 16.

Crane, P.K. et al. "Glucose Levels and Risk of Dementia." *N Engl J Med* 2013 August 8; 369: 540.

DeFina, L.F.et al."The Association between Midlife Cardiorespiratory Fitness Levels and Later-Life Dementia: A cohort study." *Ann Intern Med* 2013 February 5; 158:162.

Estruch, R. et al. "Primary Prevention of Cardiovascular Disease with the Mediterranean Diet." *N Engl J Med* 2013 February 25; [e-pub ahead of print].

Friedemann, C. et al. "Cardiovascular Disease risk in Healthy Children and its Association with Body Mass Index: Systemic review and meta-analysis." *BMJ* 2012 September 25; 345: e 479.

Flegal, K.L. et al. "Association of All-Cause Mortality with Overweight and Obesity Using Standard Body Mass Index Categories: A Systematic Review and Meta-Analysis." *JAMA* 2013 January 2; 309: 87.

Gallagher, J.C. et al. "The Effect of Vitamin D on Calcium Absorption in Older Women." *J Clin Endocrinol Metab* 2012 October; 97: 3550.

Gerstein, H.C. "Do Lifestyle Changes Reduce Serious Outcomes in Diabetes?" *N Engl J Med* 2013 July 11; 369:189

Hooper, L. et al. "Effect of Reducing Total Fat Intake on Body Weight: Systematic Review and Meta-Analysis of Randomized Controlled Trials and Cohort Studies." *BMJ* 2012 December 6; 345: e7666.

Hunter, G.R. et al. "Combined Aerobic and Strength Training and Energy Expenditure in Older Women." *Medical Science and Sports Exercise.* 2013 July; 45: 1386.

Hurt, R.D. et al. "Myocardial Infarction and Sudden Cardiac Death in Olmsted County, Minnesota, before and after Smoke-Free Workplace Laws." *Arch Intern Med* 2012 November 26; 172:1635.

Kokkinos, P.F. et al. "Interactive Effects of Fitness and Statin Treatment on Mortality Risk in Veterans with Dyslipidemia: A Cohort Study." *Lancet* 2012 November 28; [e-pub ahead of print].

Larsson, S.C. "Are Calcium Supplements harmful to cardiovascular Disease?" *JAMA Intern Med* 2013 February 4; [e-pub ahead of print].

Ortega, F.B. et al. Muscular Strength in Male adolescents and Premature Deaths: Cohort study of one million participants." *BMJ* 2012 November 20; 345: e7279.

Rizzuto, D.et al."Lifestyle, Social Factors, and Survival after Age 75: Population based study." *BMJ* 2012 August 30; 345: e 5568.

Rong, Y. et al. "Egg Consumption and Risk of Coronary Heart Disease and Stroke: Dose-response meta-analysis of prospective cohort studies." *BMJ* 2013 January 7; 346: e 8539.

Te Morenga, L. et al. Dietary Sugars and Body Weight: Systemic review and mea-analysis of randomized controlled trials and cohort studies." *BMJ* 2013 January 15; 346:e7492.

Uthman, Q.A. et al. "Exercise for Lower Limb Osteoarthritis: Systematic Review Incorporporating Trial Sequential Analysis and Network Meta-Analysis." *BMJ* 2013 September 20; 347:5555.

OTHER WORKS CITED

American Academy of Family Physicians. 'Information from Your Family Doctor: Keeping Your Heart Healthy Through Good Nutrition and Exercise,' January 15, 2006, *American Family Physician.*

The Journal of Nutrition, (Family Practice News – January 15, 2009).

Stutman, Fred, *Dr. Walk's Diet & Fitness Newsletter.* Medical Manor Books. Philadelphia, March 20

Exercise and Dementia, Eds. *Annals of Internal Medicine.* 2006 (144:73-81, 135-136).

Family Practice News – January 15, 2009), *Journal of Nutrition,*

Fitness in Adolescents and Young Males, Eds. *Journal American Medical Association,* December 21, 2005, (Vol. 294, No. 23, 2981-2988).

Journal of Nutrition, Eds, Fruits & Vegetables Reduce Incidence of Strokes. (*Family Practice News* - January 15, 2009).

Dr. Emilio Ros, Walnuts Reduce Coronary Artery Disease. *Journal of Circulation,* 2012. The Hospital Clinic of Barcelona, Spain.

Edward Colimore, *The Philadelphia Inquirer's Walking Tour of Historic Philadelphia* (Philadelphia Inquirer's Walking Tours of Historic Philadelphia) Camino Books, (February 28, 2007)

Doug Gelbert, *A Walking Tour of Philadelphia - Old City, Pennsylvania* (Look Up, America!) [Kindle Edition] Cruden Bay Books (May 23, 2009)

Roslyn F. Brenner, *Philadelphia's Outdoor Art: A Walking Tour* Camino Books; 2 edition (May 2002)

Lauran and Carrie Havranek, *Frommer's Philadelphia and the Amish Country* (Frommer's Complete Guides) Frommers; 16th edition (May 31, 2011)

John Gattuso, *Insight City Guide: Philadelphia. Long Island City:* Langenscheidt Publishers, 2007.

Richard Varr, *Eyewitness Travel: Philadelphia and the Pennsylvania Dutch Country.* New York: DK Publishing, Inc., 2007

APPENDIX
FAT & FIBER COUNTER

SOURCES OF INFORMATION

- United States Department of Agriculture
- Center for Science and Public Interest
- Food Manufacturers, Processors and Distributors
- Bowes and Church's Food Values of Portions Commonly Used (Pennington and Church, 17th Ed.)
- Scientific Journals and Publications
- Author Extrapolations

INTERPRETING FOOD LABELS

- Sugar Free: Less than ½ gram sugar per serving
- Calorie Free: No more than 5 calories per serving
- Salt Free: Less than 5 milligrams of sodium per serving
- Low Sodium: No more than 140 milligrams of sodium per serving
- Fat Free: Less than ½ gram fat per serving
- Low-fat: No more than 3 grams fat per serving
- Reduced fat: At least 25% less fat than comparison food
- Low Saturated Fat: No more than 1 gram saturated fat per serving
- Reduced Saturated Fat: No more than 50% saturated fat of comparison food
- Light: ½ the fat in or ⅓ fewer calories than the regular version of a similar food

239

BREAD AND FLOUR

Item	Serving	Tot. Fat (g)	Sat. Fat (g)	Chol. (mg)	Fiber (g)
Bagel, Plain	1 medium	1.1	0.2	0	2
Bagel, Cinnamon Raisin	1 medium	1.2	0.2	0	2
Barley Flour	1 cup	0.5	1.3	0	3
Biscuit					
Plain	1 medium	6.6	1.9	3	1
Buttermilk	1 medium	5.8	0.9	2	1
From Mix	1 medium	4.3	1.2	3	1
Bread					
Cracked Wheat	1 slice	1.0	0.2	0	1
French/Vienna	1 slice	1.0	0.2	0	1
Italian	1 slice	0.5	0.1	0	1
Matzoh	1 piece	0.5	0.1	0	0
Mixed Grain	1 slice	0.9	0.2	0	2
Multigrain, "Lite"	1 slice	0.5	0.0	2	3
Pita, Plain	1 large	0.7	0.1	0	2
Pita, Whole Wheat	1 large	1.2	0.3	0	4
Pumpernickel	1 slice	0.8	0.0	0	2
Raisin	1 slice	1.1	0.3	0	1
Rye	1 slice	0.9	0.2	0	2
Sourdough	1 slice	0.8	0.2	0	1
Wheat, Commercial	1 slice	1.1	0.3	0	2
Wheat, "Lite"	1 slice	0.5	0.1	0	3
White, Commercial	1 slice	1.0	0.2	0	0
White, "Lite"	1 slice	0.5	0.1	0	1
Whole Wheat, Commercial	1 slice	1.2	0.3	0	3
Bread Crumbs	1 cup	1.5	1.3	0	2
Breadsticks	2 small	0.5	0.2	0	0
Bulgar	½ cup	2.0	0.3	0	5.2
Cornbread	1 piece	5.5	2.0	12	1.5
Cornmeal, Dry	½ cup	2.3	0.3	0	6
Cornstarch	1 T	0.0	0.0	0	0
Crackers					
Cheese	5 pieces	4.9	1.6	4	0
Cheese Nips	13 crackers	3.2	1.2	3	0
Cheese w/Peanut Bttr	2 oz. Pkg.	13.5	2.9	7	1
Goldfish, Any Flavor	12 crackers	2.0	0.7	1	0

Item	Serving	Tot. Fat (g)	Sat. Fat (g)	Chol. (mg)	Fiber (g)
Crackers (continued)					
Graham	2 squares	1.3	0.4	0	0
Harvest Wheats	4 crackers	3.6	1.1	0	1
Melba Toast	1 piece	0.2	0.0	0	0
Oyster	15 crackers	2.1	0.3	0	0
Rice Cakes	1 piece	0.2	0.2	0	0
Ritz	3 crackers	3.0	3.0	1	0
Ritz Cheese	3 crackers	3.9	3.9	2	0
Ryekrisp, Plain	2 crackers	0.2	0.2	0	2
Ryekrisp, Sesame	2 crackers	1.4	1.4	0	3
Saltines	2 crackers	0.7	0.7	0	0
Sesame Wafers	3 crackers	3.0	3.0	0	0
Snackwell's Wheat	5 crackers	0.0	0.0	0	1
Sociables	6 crackers	3.0	3.0	0	0
Soda	5 crackers	1.9	1.9	0	0
Tsted w/Peanut Butter	1.5 oz. Pkg.	10.5	10.5	2	0
Triscuit	2 crackers	1.6	1.6	0	1
Vegetable Thins	7 crackers	4.0	4.0	0	0
Wheat Thins	4 crackers	1.5	1.5	0	0
Wheat w/Cheese	1.5 oz. Pkg.	10.9	10.9	1	0
Crepe	1 medium	12.5	12.5	37	0
Croissant	1 medium	11.5	11.5	30	1
Croutons, Commercial	¼ cup	1.8	1.8	0	1
Danish Pastry	1 medium	19.3	19.3	30	1
Doughnut					
Cake	(1) 2 oz.	16.2	16.2	24	1
Yeast	(1) 2 oz.	13.3	13.3	21	1
English Muffin					
Plain	1	1.1	1.1	0	1
w/Raisins	1	1.2	1.2	0	1
Whole Wheat	1	2.0	2.0	0	2
Flour					
Buckwheat	1 cup	3.0	3.0	0	8
Rice	1 cup	1.3	1.3	0	3
Rye	1 cup	2.2	2.2	0	11
Soy	1 cup	16.0	16.0	0	4
White, All Purpose	1 cup	1.2	1.2	0	4
Whole Wheat	1 cup	2.3	2.3	0	12

BREAD AND FLOUR (CONTINUED)

Item	Serving	Tot. Fat (g)	Sat. Fat (g)	Chol. (mg)	Fiber (g)
French Toast					
Frzn Variety	1 slice	6.0	6.0	54	0
Hmde	1 slice	10.7	10.7	75	1
Funnel Cake	4 in. diam.	12.8	12.8	48	1
Muffins					
Banana Nut	1 medium	5.0	2.2	20	2
Blueberry, From Mix	1 medium	5.1	1.1	9	1
Bran, Hmde	1 medium	5.8	1.2	16	3
Corn	1 medium	4.8	0.9	18	2
White, Plain	1 medium	5.4	1.1	12	1
Pancakes					
Blueberry, From Mix	3 medium	15.0	4.3	80	4
Buckwheat, From Mix	3 medium	12.3	3.9	75	3
Buttermilk, From Mix	3 medium	10.0	3.2	80	2
"Lite," From Mix	3 medium	2.0	0.6	20	5
Whole Wht, From Mix	3 medium	3.0	1.0	30	6
Phyllo Dough	2 oz.	6.4	0.5	0	1
Pie Crust, Plain	⅛ pie	8.0	1.9	0	0
Popover	1	5.0	2.6	51	0
Rolls					
Crescent	1	5.6	2.8	6	1
Croissant	1 small	6.0	3.5	21	0
French	1	0.4	0.1	0	1
Hamburger	1	3.0	0.8	1	1
Hard	1	1.2	0.3	1	1
Hot Dog	1	2.1	0.5	1	1
Kaiser	1 medium	2.0	0.5	0	0
Raisin	1 large	1.9	0.5	0	1
Rye, Dark	1	1.6	0.1	0	2
Rye, Light, Hard	1	1.0	0.1	0	2
Sandwich	1	3.1	0.4	2	1
Sesame Seed	1	2.1	0.6	1	1
Sourdough	1	1.0	0.0	0	1
Submarine/Hoagie	1 medium	3.0	0.8	3	2
Wheat	1	1.7	0.4	0	1
White, Commercial	1	2.2	1.0	1	0
Whole Wheat	1	1.1	0.2	1	3

Item	Serving	Tot. Fat (g)	Sat. Fat (g)	Chol. (mg)	Fiber (g)
Scone	1	5.5	1.5	28	1
Soft Pretzel	1 medium	1.5	0.7	2	1.5
Stuffing					
Bread, From Mix	½ cup	12.2	6.0	0	0
Cornbread, From Mix	½ cup	4.8	2.5	43	0
Stove Top	½ cup	9.0	5.0	21	0
Sweet Roll, Iced	1 medium	7.9	2.1	20	1
Toaster Pastry	1	5.0	0.8	0	0
Tortilla					
Corn (Unfried)	1 medium	1.1	0.2	0	1
Flour	1 medium	2.5	1.1	0	1
Turnover, Fruit Filled	1	15.0	3.7	0	1
Waffle					
Frozen	1 medium	3.2	0.8	11	1
Hmde	1 medium	9.5	4.1	50	1
From Mix	1 medium	8.5	3.0	48	1

CEREALS

Item	Serving	Tot. Fat (g)	Sat. Fat (g)	Chol. (mg)	Fiber (g)
All Bran	⅓ cup	0.5	0.1	0	10
Apple Jacks	1 cup	0.1	0.0	0	1
Bran, 100%	½ cup	1.9	0.3	0	9
Bran Chex	1 cup	1.2	0.2	0	9
Bran Flakes, 40%	1 cup	0.7	0.1	0	6
Cheerios	1 cup	1.6	0.3	0	2
Cocoa Krispies	1 cup	0.5	0.2	0	0
Corn Chex	1 cup	0.1	0.0	0	1
Cornflakes	1 cup	0.1	0.0	0	1
Cracklin' Oat Bran	⅓ cup	2.7	1.3	0	3
Cream of Wheat w/o Fat	½ cup	0.3	0.0	0	0
Crispix	1 cup	0.0	0.0	0	1
Fiber One	1 cup	2.0	0.4	0	13
Frosted Bran, Kellogg's	¾ cup	0.0	0.0	0	3
Frosted Mini-Wheats	4 biscuits	0.3	0.0	0	1
Fruit and Fiber w/Dates, Raisins					
Walnuts	⅔ cup	2.0	0.3	0	5
w/Peaches, Almonds	⅔ cup	2.0	0.3	0	5

CEREALS (CONTINUED)

Item	Serving	Tot. Fat (g)	Sat. Fat (g)	Chol. (mg)	Fiber (g)
Fruitful Bran	⅔ cup	0.0	0.0	0	5
Fruit Loops	1 cup	0.5	0.0	0	1
Golden Grahams	¾ cup	1.1	0.1		1
Granola					
Commercial Brands	⅓ cup	4.9	1.8	0	3
Low-Fat, Kellogg's	⅓ cup	2.0	0.0	0	2
Grapenut Flakes	1 cup	0.4	0.2	0	2
Grapenuts	¼ cup	0.1	0.0	0	2
Life, Plain Or Cinn.	1 cup	2.5	0.5	0	4
Mueslix, Kellogg's	½ cup	1.0	0.8	0	5
Nutri-Grain, Kellogg's					
Almond Raisin	⅔ cup	2.0	0.4	0	3
Raisin Bran	1 cup	1.0	0.1	0	5
Wheat	⅔ cup	0.3	0.0	0	3
Oat Bran, Cooked Cereal					
w/o Added Fat	½ cup	0.5	0.1	0	2
Oats					
Instant	1 packet	1.7	0.2	0	1
w/o Added Fat	½ cup	1.2	0.2	0	1
Product 19	1 cup	0.2	0.0	0	1
Puffed Rice	1 cup	0.2	0.0	0	1
Puffed Wheat	1 cup	0.1	0.0	0	1
Raisin Bran	1 cup	0.8	0.1	0	5
Rice Chex	1 cup	0.1	0.0	0	1
Rice Krispies	1 cup	0.2	0.0	0	0
Shredded Wheat	1 cup	0.3	0.0	0	2
Special K	1 cup	0.1	0.0	0	0
Sugar Frosted Flakes	1 cup	0.5	0.1	0	1
Total	1 cup	0.7	0.1	0	2
Total Raisin Bran	1 cup	1.0	0.1	0	5
Wheat Chex	1 cup	1.2	0.2	0	6
Wheaties	1 cup	0.5	0.1	0	2

DAIRY PRODUCTS (CHEESES)

Item	Serving	Tot. Fat (g)	Sat. Fat (g)	Chol. (mg)	Fiber (g)
American					
Processed	1 oz.	8.9	5.6	27	0
Reduced Calorie	1 oz.	2.0	1.0	12	0
Blue	1 oz.	8.2	5.3	21	0
Borden's Fat Free	1 oz.	<0.5	<0.3	<5	0
Borden's Lite Line	1 oz.	2.0	<1.0	NA	0
Caraway	1 oz.	8.3	5.4	30	0
Cheddar	1 oz.	9.2	5.0	26	0
Cheese Sauce	¼ cup	9.8	4.3	20	0
Cheese Spread, Kraft	1 oz.	6.0	3.8	16	0
Cheez Whiz	1 oz.	6.0	3.1	16	0
Cottage Cheese					
1% Fat	½ cup	1.2	0.8	5	0
2% Fat	½ cup	2.2	1.4	10	0
Creamed	½ cup	5.1	3.2	17	0
Cream Cheese					
Kraft Free	1 oz. (2T)	0.0	0.0	5	0
Lite	1 oz. (2T)	6.6	4.2	20	0
Regular	1 oz. (2T)	9.9	6.2	31	0
Edam	1 oz.	7.9	5.0	25	0
Feta	1 oz.	6.0	4.2	25	0
Gouda	1 oz.	7.8	5.0	32	0
Jarlsberg	1 oz.	6.9	4.2	16	0
Kraft American Singles	1 oz.	7.5	4.3	25	0
Kraft Free Singles	1 oz.	0.0	0.0	5	0
Kraft Light Singles	1 oz.	4.0	2.0	15	0
Light N'lively Singles	1 oz.	4.0	2.0	15	0
Monterey Jack	1 oz.	8.6	5.0	30	0
Mozzarella					
Part Skim	1 oz.	4.5	2.4	16	0
Whole Milk	1 oz.	6.1	3.7	22	0
Muenster	1 oz.	8.5	5.4	27	0
Parmesan					
Grated	1 T	1.5	1.0	4	0
Hard	1 oz.	7.3	4.7	19	0
Pimento Cheese Spread	1 oz.	8.9	5.6	27	0

DAIRY PRODUCTS (CHEESES) CONTINUED

Item	Serving	Tot. Fat (g)	Sat. Fat (g)	Chol. (mg)	Fiber (g)
Provolone	1 oz.	7.6	4.8	20	0
Ricotta					
"Lite" Reduced Fat	½ cup	4.0	2.4	15	0
Part Skim	½ cup	9.8	6.1	38	0
Whole Milk	½ cup	16.1	10.3	63	0
Romano	1 oz.	7.6	4.9	29	0
Roquefort	1 oz.	7.8	5.0	24	0
Swiss					
Alpine Lace	1 oz.	1.5	0.5	5	0
Sliced	1 oz.	7.8	5.0	26	0
Velveeta	1 oz.	7.0	4.0	20	0
Velveeta Light	1 oz.	4.0	2.0	15	0

EGGS

Item	Serving	Tot. Fat (g)	Sat. Fat (g)	Chol. (mg)	Fiber (g)
Boiled-Poached	1	5.6	1.6	213	0
Fried w/ ½ Tbs Margarine	1 large	7.6	2.7	240	0
Omelet					
2 Oz. Cheese, 3 Egg	1	37.0	12.3	480	0
Plain, 3 Egg	1	21.3	5.2	430	0
Spanish, 2 Egg	1	18.0	5.9	375	1
Scrambled w/Milk	1 large	8.0	2.8	214	0
Substitute, Frzn	¼ cup	0.0	0.0	0	0
White	1 large	0.0	0.0	0	0
Yolk	1 large	5.6	1.6	213	0

MILK AND YOGURT

Item	Serving	Tot. Fat (g)	Sat. Fat (g)	Chol. (mg)	Fiber (g)
Buttermilk					
1% Fat	1 cup	2.2	1.3	9	0
Dry	1 T	0.4	0.2	5	0
Chocolate Milk					
2% Fat	1 cup	5.0	3.1	17	0
Whole	1 cup	8.5	5.3	30	0
Evaporated Milk					
Skim	½ cup	0.4	0.0	0	0
Whole	½ cup	9.5	5.8	37	0
Hot Cocoa					
Mix w/Water	1 cup	3.0	0.7	5	0
w/Skim Milk	1 cup	2.0	0.9	12	0
w/Whole Milk	1 cup	9.1	5.6	33	0
Low-fat Milk					
½% Fat	1 cup	1.0	4.0	10	0
1% Fat	1 cup	2.6	1.6	10	0
2% Fat	1 cup	4.7	2.9	18	0
Milkshake					
Choc. Thick	1 cup	6.1	3.8	24	1
Vanilla, Thick	1 cup	6.9	4.3	27	0
Skim Milk					
Liquid	1 cup	0.4	0.3	4	0
Nonfat Dry Powder	¼ cup	0.2	0.2	6	0
Whole Milk					
3.5% Fat	1 cup	8.2	5.0	34	0
Dry Powder	¼ cup	8.6	5.4	31	0
Yogurt					
Frzn, Low-fat	½ cup	3.0	2.0	10	0
Frzn, Nonfat	½ cup	0.2	0.0	0	0
Fruit Flavored, Low-fat	1 cup	2.6	0.1	10	0
Plain Yogurt					
Low-fat	1 cup	3.5	2.3	14	0
Skim (Nonfat)	1 cup	0.4	0.3	4	0
Whole Milk	1 cup	7.4	4.8	29	0

DESSERTS

Item	Serving	Tot. Fat (g)	Sat. Fat (g)	Chol. (mg)	Fiber (g)
Apple Betty	½ cup	13.3	2.7	0	3
Baklava	1 piece	29.2	7.2	7	2
Brownie					
Choc., Plain	1	5.0	1.5	14	0
Choc. w/Frosting	1	9.0	1.5	20	1
Choc. w/Nuts	1	7.3	1.8	10	1
Cake					
Angel Food	⅛ cake	0.1	0.0	0	0
Banana	⅛ cake	14.5	2.5	50	1
Black Forest	⅛ cake	15.0	2.0	50	1
Carrot w/Frosting	⅛ cake	18.0	3.6	53	3
Choc. w/Frosting	⅛ cake	16.0	4.0	77	2
Coconut w/Frosting	⅛ cake	17.0	5.4	51	2
Coffee Cake	⅛ cake	6.1	1.0	42	1
Devil's Food, "Light" From Mix	⅛ cake	2.8	1.1	42	0
German Choc. w/ Frosting	⅛ cake	17.0	4.1	72	2
Gingerbread	⅛ cake	2.6	0.9	1.3	0
Lemon Chiffon	⅛ cake	3.0	0.7	3	0
Marble w/Frosting	⅛ cake	15.0	2.5	62	1
Pound	⅛ cake	8.2	4.0	50	1
Spice w/Frosting	⅛ cake	10.2	2.8	48	1
Sponge	⅛ cake	2.0	0.5	50	0
White w/Frosting	⅛ cake	13.1	3.0	30	1
White, "Light," From Mix	⅛ cake	2.6	0.5	15	0
Yellow, "Light," From Mix	⅛ cake	3.0	1.2	35	0
Yellow w/Frosting	⅛ cake	14.0	4.0	50	1
Cheesecake, Traditional	⅛ pie	22.0	10.4	36	0
Cobbler					
w/Biscuit Topping	½ cup	6.0	1.7	2	3
w/Pie-Crust Topping	½ cup	9.3	3.6	5	3
Cookies					
Animal	15 cookies	4.7	1.2	0	0

Item	Serving	Tot. Fat (g)	Sat. Fat (g)	Chol. (mg)	Fiber (g)
Cookies (continued)					
Chantilly, Pepperidge Farm	1	2.0	1.0	<5	0
Choc.	1	3.3	1.0	6	0
Choc. Chip Hmde	1	3.7	2.0	8	0
Choc. Chip, Pepperidge Farm	1	2.5	1.4	<5	0
Choc. Sandwich (Oreo Type)	1	2.1	0.4	0	0
Entenmann's Fat-Free	2	0.0	0.0	0	0
Fat-Free Newtons	1	0.0	0.0	0	0
Fig Bar	1	1.0	0.2	0	1
Fig Newtons	1	1.0	0.3	0	0
Gingersnap	1	1.6	0.3	0	0
Graham Cracker, Choc. Covered	1	3.1	0.9	0	0
Macaroon, Coconut	1	3.4	1.3	0	0
Oatmeal	1	3.2	0.6	0	0
Oatmeal Raisin	1	3.0	0.8	0	0
Peanut Butter	1	3.2	1.0	6	1
Rice Krispie Bar	1	0.9	0.3	0	0
Shortbread	1	2.3	0.4	2	0
Cupcake					
Choc. w/Icing	1	5.5	2.1	22	1
Yellow w/Icing	1	6.0	2.3	23	1
Custard, Baked	½ cup	6.9	3.4	123	0
Date Bar	1 bar	2.0	0.7	2	1
Dumpling, Fruit	1 piece	15.1	5.5	8	2
Éclair (With Choc. Icing & Custard)	1 small	15.4	5.7	115	0
Fruitcake	1 piece	6.2	1.4	11	1
Fruit Ice, Italian	½ cup	0.0	0.0	0	0
Fudgesicle	1 bar	0.4	0.2	3	1
Granola Bar	1 bar	6.8	1.5	0	1
Ice Cream					
Choc. (10% Fat)	½ cup	7.3	4.5	23	1
Choc. (16% Fat)	½ cup	17.0	8.9	44	0
Dietetic, Sugar-Free	½ cup	3.5	1.3	27	0
Vanilla Soft Serve	½ cup	11.3	6.4	76	0

DESSERTS (CONTINUED)

Item	Serving	Tot. Fat (g)	Sat. Fat (g)	Chol. (mg)	Fiber (g)
Ice Cream (continued)					
Strawberry (10% Fat)	½ cup	6.0	4.0	28	0
Vanilla (10% Fat)	½ cup	7.0	5.4	28	0
Vanilla (16% Fat)	½ cup	11.9	7.4	44	0
Ice Cream Bar					
Choc. Coated	1 bar	11.5	10.0	23	0
Toffee Crunch	1 bar	10.2	7.0	9	1
Ice Cream Cake Roll	1 slice	6.9	4.0	52	0
Ice Cream Cone (Cone Only)	1 medium	0.3	0.1	0	0
Ice Cream Drumstick	1	10.0	4.1	14	1
Ice Cream Sandwich	1	8.3	4.4	12	0
Ice Milk					
Choc.	½ cup	2.0	1.3	9	0
Soft Serve, All Flavors	½ cup	2.3	1.4	7	0
Strawberry	½ cup	2.5	1.2	7	0
Vanilla	½ cup	2.8	1.5	8	0
Jello	½ cup	0.0	0.0	0	0
Ladyfinger	1	2.0	0.5	80	0
Lemon Bars	1 bar	3.2	7.0	13	0
Mousse, Choc.	½ cup	15.5	8.7	124	1
Napoleon	1 piece	5.3	2.6	10	0
Pie					
Apple	⅛ pie	16.9	2.3	3	3
Banana Cream Or Custard	⅛ pie	14.0	10.0	35	1
Blueberry	⅛ pie	17.3	4.0	0	3
Boston Cream Pie	⅛ pie	10.0	3.1	20	1
Cherry	⅛ pie	18.1	5.0	0	2
Choc. Cream	⅛ pie	13.0	4.5	15	3
Coconut Cream Or Custard	⅛ pie	19.0	7.0	80	1
Key Lime	⅛ pie	19.0	6.8	10	1
Lemon Chiffon	⅛ pie	13.5	3.7	15	1
Lemon Meringue, Traditional	⅛ pie	13.1	5.1	50	1
Peach	⅛ pie	17.7	4.6	3	3

Item	Serving	Tot. Fat (g)	Sat. Fat (g)	Chol. (mg)	Fiber (g)
Pie (continued)					
Pecan	⅛ pie	23.0	3.5	100	2
Pumpkin	⅛ pie	16.8	5.7	109	
Raisin	⅛ pie	12.9	3.1	0	1
Rhubarb	⅛ pie	17.1	4.5	2	3
Strawberry	⅛ pie	9.1	4.5	2	1
Sweet Potato	⅛ pie	18.2	6.0	70	2
Pie Tart, Fruit Filled	1	18.7	6.2	23	2
Popsicle	1 bar	0.0	0.0	0	0
Pudding					
Any Flavor Except Choc.	½ cup	4.3	2.5	70	0
Bread w/Raisins	½ cup	7.4	2.9	79	1
Choc. w/Whole Milk	½ cup	5.7	3.1	17	1
From Mix w/Skim Milk	½ cup	0.0	0.0	0	0
Rice w/Whole Milk	½ cup	4.4	2.5	16	1
Sugar Free Varieties	½ cup	2.2	1.4	10	0
Tapioca, w/2% Milk	½ cup	2.4	1.5	8	0
Pudding Pop, Frzn	1 bar	2.0	1.0	2	0
Sherbert	½ cup	1.0	0.5	7	0
Souffle, Choc.	½ cup	3.9	1.4	42	0
Strudel, Fruit	½ cup	1.2	0.1	2	1
Toppings					
Butterscotch/Caramel	3 T	0.1	0.0	0	0
Cherry	3 T	0.1	0.0	0	0
Choc. Fudge	2 T	4.0	2.0	0	0
Choc. Syrup, Hershey	2 T	0.4	0.2	0	0
Marshmallow	3 T	0.0	0.0	0	0
Milk Choc. Fudge	2 T	5.0	2.9	5	0
Pecans In Syrup	3 T	2.8	1.1	0	2
Pineapple	3 T	0.2	0.0	0	0
Strawberry	3 T	0.1	0.0	0	0
Whipped Topping					
Aerosol	¼ cup	3.6	1.4	0	0
From Mix	¼ cup	2.0	1.2	4	0
Frzn, Tub	¼ cup	4.8	3.6	0	0
Non-Fat	1 T	0.0	0.0	0	0

DESSERTS (CONTINUED)

Item	Serving	Tot. Fat (g)	Sat. Fat (g)	Chol. (mg)	Fiber (g)
Whipping Cream					
Heavy, Fluid	1 T	5.6	3.5	21	0
Light, Fluid	1 T	4.6	2.9	17	0
Turnover, Fruit Filled	1	19.3	5.4	2	1
Yogurt, Frozen					
Low-fat	½ cup	1.9	1.2	10	0
Nonfat	½ cup	0.0	0.0	0	0

CANDY

Item	Serving	Tot. Fat (g)	Sat. Fat (g)	Chol. (mg)	Fiber (g)
Butterscotch					
Candy	6 pieces	1.3	0.4	0	0
Chips	1 oz.	8.3	6.8	0	0
Candied Fruit					
Apricot	1 oz.	0.1	0.0	0	1
Cherry	1 oz.	0.1	0.0	0	1
Citrus Peel	1 oz.	0.1	0.0	0	1
Figs	1 oz.	0.1	0.0	0	2
Candy Bar (Average)	1 oz.	8.5	4.5	5	1
Caramels					
Plain Or Choc. w/Nuts	1 oz.	4.6	2.2	10	0
Plain Or Choc. w/o Nuts	1 oz.	3.0	1.3	9	0
Choc.-Covered Cherries	1 oz.	4.9	2.9	1	1
Choc.-Covered Cream Center	1 oz.	4.9	2.6	1	1
Choc.-Covered Mint Patty	1 small	1.5	0.8	8	0
Choc.-Covered Peanuts	1 oz.	11.7	4.6	8	2
Choc.-Covered Raisins	1 oz.	4.9	2.9	3	1
Choc. Kisses	6 pieces	9.0	5.0	6	1
Choc. Stars	6 pieces	8.1	4.7	5	12
Cracker Jack	1 cup	3.3	0.4	0	0
English Toffee	1 oz.	2.8	1.7	5	
Fudge					
Choc.	1 oz.	3.4	1.5	1	0
Choc. w/Nuts	1 oz.	4.9	1.2	1	0

Item	Serving	Tot. Fat (g)	Sat. Fat (g)	Chol. (mg)	Fiber (g)
Gumdrops	28 pieces	0.2	0.0	0	0
Gummy Bears	1 oz.	0.1	0.0	0	0
Hard Candy	6 pieces	0.3	0.0	0	0
Jelly Beans	1 oz.	0.0	0.0	0	0
Licorice	1 oz.	0.1	0.0	0	0
Life Savers	5 pieces	0.1	0.0	0	0
M&M's					
Choc. Only	1 oz.	5.6	2.4	3	1
Peanut	1 oz.	7.8	2.4	4	1
Malted-Milk Balls	1 oz.	7.1	4.2	3	1
Marshmallow	1 large	0.0	0.0	0	0
Mints	14 pieces	0.6	0.0	0	0
Peanut Brittle	1 oz.	7.7	1.2	0	1
Peanut Butter Cups	1 oz.	9.2	3.6	3	1
Peppermint Pattie	1 oz.	3.0	2.0	0	<1
Raisinettes	1 oz.	5.5	3.0	4	0
Reese's Pieces	1.7 oz. pkg.	13.0	5.2	2	0
Sour Balls	1 oz.	0.0	0.0	0	0
Taffy	1 oz.	1.5	0.4	0	0
Tootsie Roll Pop	1 oz.	0.6	0.2	0	0
Tootsie Roll	1 oz.	2.3	0.6	0	1

FATS

Item	Serving	Tot. Fat (g)	Sat. Fat (g)	Chol. (mg)	Fiber (g)
Bacon Fat	1 T	14.0	6.4	0	0
Beef, Separable Fat	1 oz.	23.3	6.0	0	0
Butter					
Solid	1 t	3.8	2.4	0	0
Whipped	1 t	2.6	1.6	0	0
Butter Buds, Liquid	2 T	0.0	0.0	0	0
Butter Sprinkles	½ t	0.0	0.0	0	0
Chicken Fat, Raw	1 T	12.8	3.8	0	0
Cream					
Light	1 T	2.9	1.8	0	0
Medium (25% Fat)	1 T	3.8	2.3	0	0
Whipping, Light	1T	4.6	2.9	0	0

FATS (CONTINUED)

Item	Serving	Tot. Fat (g)	Sat. Fat (g)	Chol. (mg)	Fiber (g)
Cream, Substitute					
Liquid/Frzn	½ fl. oz.	1.5	1.4	0	0
Powdered	1 T	0.7	0.7	0	0
Half & Half	1 T	1.7	1.1	0	0
Margarine					
Liquid Or Soft Tub	1 t	3.8	0.6	0	0
Reduced Calorie Tub	1 t	2.0	0.3	0	0
Solid (Corn), Stick	1 t	3.8	0.6	0	0
Fat-Free Tub	1 t	0.0	0.0	0	0
Mayonnaise					
Fat-Free	1 T	0.0	0.0	0	0
Reduced Calorie	1 T	5.0	0.7	0	0
Regular	1 T	12.0	1.3	0	0
No-Stick Spray (Pam, etc.)	2-sec spray	0.9	0.2	0	0
Oil					
Canola	1 T	13.6	1.0	0	0
Corn	1 T	13.6	1.7	0	0
Olive	1 T	13.5	1.8	0	0
Safflower	1 T	13.6	1.2	0	0
Soybean	1 T	13.6	2.0	0	0
Pork Fat (Lard)	1 T	12.8	5.0	0	0
Sandwich Spread (Miracle Whip Type)	1 T	4.9	0.7	0	0
Shortening, Vegetable	1 T	12.8	3.2	0	0
Sour Cream					
Cultured	1 T	3.0	1.9	0	0
Fat-Free	1 T	0.0	0.0	0	0
Half & Half, Cultured	1 T	1.8	1.1	0	0
Low-fat	1 T	1.8	1.1	0	0

FISH (ALL BAKED/BROILED W/O ADDED FAT UNLESS OTHERWISE NOTED)

Item	Serving	Tot. Fat (g)	Sat. Fat (g)	Chol. (mg)	Fiber (g)
Abalone, Canned	3 oz.	5.2	0.3	80	0
Anchovy, Canned In Oil	3 fillets	1.2	0.3	10	0
Bass					
Freshwater	3 oz.	4.5	0.9	60	0
Saltwater, Black	3 oz.	1.0	0.2	50	0
Saltwater, Striped	3 oz.	2.3	0.6	70	0
Bluefish					
Cooked	3 oz.	5.2	1.3	50	0
Fried	3 oz.	12.6	2.7	59	0
Butterfish					
Gulf	3 oz.	2.6	0.7	60	0
Northern	3 oz.	10.0	1.9	49	0
Carp	3 oz.	6.0	1.4	72	0
Catfish	3 oz.	3.0	0.7	60	0
Catfish, Breaded & Fried	3 oz.	13.0	2.9	75	1
Caviar, Sturgeon, Granular	1 t	1.5	0.4	47	0
Clams					
Canned, Solids & Liquid	½ cup	0.7	0.1	25	0
Meat Only	5 large	1.0	0.2	42	0
Soft, Raw	4 large	0.8	0.1	29	0
Cod					
Canned	3 oz.	0.6	0.2	45	0
Cooked	3 oz.	0.6	0.2	40	0
Dried, Salted	3 oz.	2.0	0.5	129	0
Crab					
Canned	½ cup	0.9	0.1	60	0
Deviled	3 oz.	10.0	3.5	40	0
Fried, Cake	3 oz.	18.0	4.1	170	0
Crab, Alaska King	3 oz.	1.2	0.2	53	0
Crab Cake	3 oz.	10.6	1.2	100	0
Crayfish, Freshwater	3 oz.	1.2	0.2	115	0
Croaker					
Atlantic	3 oz.	3.0	1.0	60	0
White	3 oz.	0.6	0.3	60	0
Dolphin Fish	3 oz.	0.8	0.2	72	0

FISH (CONTINUED)

Item	Serving	Tot. Fat (g)	Sat. Fat (g)	Chol. (mg)	Fiber (g)
Fillets, Frzn					
Batter Dipped	2 pieces	20.0	4.0	40	1
Breaded	2 pieces	18.0	3.0	35	1
Fish Cakes, Frzn, Fried	3 oz.	13.8	3.9	102	2
Flounder/Sole	3 oz.	0.4	0.2	30	0
Gefilte Fish	3 oz.	2.0	0.5	50	1
Grouper	3 oz.	1.2	0.3	45	0
Haddock					
Cooked	3 oz.	0.5	0.1	50	0
Fried	3 oz.	14.0	3.7	60	0
Halibut	3 oz.	1.0	0.5	30	0
Herring					
Canned Or Smoked	3 oz.	16.0	6.0	66	0
Cooked	3 oz.	11.0	2.0	70	0
Kingfish	3 oz.	3.0	0.8	68	0
Lobster					
Broiled With Butter	12 oz.	15.1	8.6	100	0
Steamed	3 oz.	0.5	0.1	70	0
Mackerel					
Atlantic	3 oz.	13.0	1.5	60	0
Pacific	3 oz.	12.5	1.7	55	0
Mussels, Meat Only	3 oz.	2.0	0.7	30	0
Ocean Perch					
Cooked	3 oz.	1.4	0.3	40	0
Fried	3 oz.	11.4	2.8	62	0
Octopus	3 oz.	2.0	0.4	95	0
Oysters					
Canned	3 oz.	2.0	0.8	54	0
Fried	3 oz.	13.7	3.2	83	0
Raw	5 – 8 med	1.8	0.6	54	0
Perch, Freshwater, Yellow	3 oz.	0.8	0.4	80	0
Pike					
Blue	3 oz.	0.7	0.5	75	0
Northern	3 oz.	1.0	0.7	40	0
Walleye	3 oz.	1.0	1.0	80	0
Pompano	3 oz.	9.5	5.0	55	0

Item	Serving	Tot. Fat (g)	Sat. Fat (g)	Chol. (mg)	Fiber (g)
Rainbow Trout					
Baked/Broiled	3 oz.	5.6	1.6	70	0
Breaded, Fried	3 oz.	14.4	3.2	84	1
Red Snapper	3 oz.	1.7	0.5	35	0
Rockfish, Oven Steamed	3 oz.	2.3	0.8	40	0
Roughy, Orange	3 oz.	2.0	0.1	20	0
Salmon					
Atlantic	3 oz.	6.2	0.9	55	0
Broiled/Baked	3 oz.	7.3	2.0	50	0
Chinook, Canned	3 oz.	7.0	2.0	50	0
Pink, Canned	3 oz.	5.0	1.3	54	0
Smoked	3 oz.	9.2	1.0	35	0
Sardines					
Atlantic, In Soy Oil	4 sardines	7.0	0.8	67	0
Skinless & Boneless	3 oz.	6.0	1.5	30	0
Scallops					
Cooked	3 oz.	1.0	0.2	30	0
Frzn, Fried	3 oz.	10.3	2.3	55	0
Steamed	3 oz.	1.2	0.2	40	0
Sea Bass, White	3 oz.	1.3	0.6	40	0
Shrimp					
Canned, Dry Pack	3 oz.	1.4	0.5	155	0
Canned, Wet Pack	3 oz.	0.6	0.3	125	0
Fried	3 oz.	10.5	0.9	120	0
Raw Or Broiled	3 oz.	1.0	0.5	150	0
Sole, Fillet	3 oz.	0.3	0.2	30	0
Squid					
Broiled	3 oz.	1.5	0.5	250	0
Fried	3 oz.	6.4	1.6	275	0
Raw	3 oz.	1.2	0.4	250	0
Sushi Or Sashimi	3 oz.	4.8	1.3	38	0
Swordfish	3 oz.	4.0	1.1	43	0
Trout					
Brook	3 oz.	3.5	0.9	60	0
Rainbow	3 oz.	7.5	1.2	85	0
Tuna					
Albacore	3 oz.	7.3	0.2	70	0
Canned, White In Oil	3 oz.	8.0	1.6	31	0

FISH (CONTINUED)

Item	Serving	Tot. Fat (g)	Sat. Fat (g)	Chol. (mg)	Fiber (g)
Tuna (continued)					
Canned, White In Water	3 oz.	1.5	0.5	25	0
Yellowfin	3 oz.	3.0	0.5	57	0
White Perch	3 oz.	3.7	0.7	65	0
Whiting	3 oz.	3.0	0.4	70	0
Yellowtail	3 oz.	5.2	0.9	75	0

FRUIT

Item	Serving	Tot. Fat (g)	Sat. Fat (g)	Chol. (mg)	Fiber (g)
Apple					
Dried	½ cup	0.1	0.0	0	5
Whole w/Peel	1 medium	0.4	0.1	0	4
Applesauce, Unsweetened	½ cup	0.1	0.0	0	2
Apricots					
Dried	5 halves	0.2	0.0	0	6
Fresh	3 medium	0.4	0.0	0	2
Avocado					
California	1 (6 oz.)	30.0	4.5	0	4
Florida	1 (11 oz.)	28.0	4.3	0	4
Blackberries					
Fresh	1 cup	0.6	0.0	0	7
Frzn, Unsweetened	1 cup	0.7	0.0	0	7
Blueberries					
Fresh	1 cup	0.6	0.0	0	5
Frzn, Unsweetened	1 cup	0.7	0.2	0	4
Boysenberries, Frzn Unsweetened	1 cup	0.4	0.0	0	6
Cantaloupe	1 cup	0.4	0.0	0	3
Cherries	½ cup	0.8	0.2	0	2
Cranberries, Fresh	1 cup	0.2	0.0	0	4
Cranberry Sauce	½ cup	0.2	0.0	0	1
Dates, Whole, Dried	½ cup	0.4	0.0	0	8
Figs					
Canned	3 figs	0.1	0.0	0	9
Dried, Uncooked	10 figs	1.1	0.4	0	10
Fresh	1 medium	0.2	0.0	0	2

Item	Serving	Tot. Fat (g)	Sat. Fat (g)	Chol. (mg)	Fiber (g)
Fruit Cocktail, Canned w/ Juice	1 cup	0.3	0.0	0	5
Fruit Roll-Up	1	0.0	0.0	0	0
Grapefruit	½ med.	0.1	0.0	0	1
Grapes, Seedless	½ cup	0.1	0.0	0	1
Guava, Fresh	1 medium	0.5	0.2	0	7
Honeydew Melon, Fresh	¼ small	0.1	0.0	0	1
Kiwi, Fresh	1 medium	0.3	0.0	0	2
Kumquat, Fresh	1 medium	0.0	0.0	0	1
Lemon, Fresh	1 medium	0.2	0.0	0	1
Lime, Fresh	1 medium	0.1	0.0	0	1
Mandarin Oranges, Canned w/Juice	½ cup	0.0	0.0	0	4
Mango, Fresh	1 medium	0.6	0.0	0	4
Melon Balls, Frzn	1 cup	0.4	0.0	0	2
Mixed Fruit					
Dried	½ cup	0.5	0.0	0	5
Frzn, Unsweetened	1 cup	0.5	0.2	0	2
Nectarine, Fresh	1 medium	0.6	0.0	0	2
Orange					
Naval, Fresh	1 medium	0.1	0.0	0	4
Valencia, Fresh	1 medium	0.4	0.0	0	4
Papaya, Fresh	1 medium	0.4	0.1	0	3
Peach					
Canned, Water Pack	1 cup	0.1	0.0	0	4
Canned In Heavy Syrup	1 cup	0.1	0.0	0	4
Canned In Light Syrup	1 cup	0.1	0.0	0	4
Fresh	1 medium	0.1	0.0	0	1
Frzn, Sweetened	1 cup	0.3	0.0	0	4
Pear					
Canned In Heavy Syrup	1 cup	0.3	0.0	0	6
Canned In Light Syrup	1 cup	0.1	0.0	0	6
Fresh	1 medium	0.7	0.0	0	5
Persimmon, Fresh	1 medium	0.1	0.0	0	3
Pineapple Pieces					
Canned, Unsweetened	1 cup	0.2	0.0	0	2
Fresh	1 cup	0.7	0.0	0	3
Plantain, Cooked, Sliced	1 cup	0.2	0.0	0	2

FRUIT (CONTINUED)

Item	Serving	Tot. Fat (g)	Sat. Fat (g)	Chol. (mg)	Fiber (g)
Plum					
Canned In Heavy Syrup	½ cup	0.1	0.0	0	4
Fresh	1 medium	0.4	0.0	0	3
Pomegranate, Fresh	1 medium	0.5	0.0	0	2
Prunes, Dried, Cooked	½ cup	0.2	0.0	0	10
Raisins					
Dark Seedless	½ cup	0.4	0.2	0	6
Golden Seedless	½ cup	0.4	0.2	0	6
Raspberries					
Fresh	1 cup	0.7	0.1	0	5
Frzn, Sweetened	1 cup	0.4	0.0	0	10
Rhubarb, Stewed, Unswetnd	1 cup	0.2	0.0	0	6
Strawberries					
Fresh	1 cup	0.6	0.0	0	3
Frzn, Sweetened	1 cup	0.3	0.0	0	3
Frzn, Unsweetened	1 cup	0.2	0.0	0	3
Tangerine, Fresh	1 medium	0.2	0.0	0	3
Watermelon, Fresh	1 cup	0.5	0.0	0	1

FRUIT JUICES

Item	Serving	Tot. Fat (g)	Sat. Fat (g)	Chol. (mg)	Fiber (g)
Apple Juice	1 cup	0.3	0.0	0	1
Apricot Nectar	1 cup	0.2	0.0	0	2
Carrot Juice	1 cup	0.4	0.0	0	2
Cranberry Juice Cocktail	1 cup	0.2	0.0	0	2
Cranberry-Apple Juice	1 cup	0.2	0.0	0	1.5
Grape Juice	1 cup	0.2	0.0	0	1
Grapefruit Juice	1 cup	0.2	0.0	0	1.5
Lemon Juice	2 T	0.0	0.0	0	0
Lime Juice	2 T	0.0	0.0	0	0
Orange Juice	1 cup	0.4	0.0	0	1
Peach Juice Or Nectar	1 cup	0.1	0.0	0	1
Pear Juice Or Nectar	1 cup	0.0	0.0	0	1
Pineapple Juice	1 cup	0.2	0.0	0	1
Prune Juice	1 cup	0.1	0.0	0	3
Tomato Juice	1 cup	0.2	0.0	0	2
V8 Juice	1 cup	0.1	0.0	0	2

LUNCH/DINNER COMBOS

Item	Serving	Tot. Fat (g)	Sat. Fat (g)	Chol. (mg)	Fiber (g)
Baked Bean w/Pork	½ cup	1.8	0.8	8	4
Beans					
Refried, Canned	½ cup	1.4	0.5	5	7
Refried, w/Fat	½ cup	13.2	5.2	12	7
Refried, Non-Fat	½ cup	0.0	0.0	0	7
Beans & Franks, Canned	1 cup	16.0	6.0	15	7
Beef & Vegetable Stew	1 cup	10.5	4.9	64	2
Beef Goulash w/Noodles	1 cup	13.9	3.6	87	2
Beef Noodle Casserole	1 cup	19.2	6.5	81	2
Beef Pot Pie	8 oz.	25.0	6.4	40	2
Beef Vegetable Stew	1 cup	10.5	5.0	64	2
Burrito					
Bean w/Cheese	1 large	11.0	5.4	26	4
Bean w/o Cheese	1 large	6.8	3.4	3	4
Beef	1 large	19.0	10.1	70	2
Cabbage Roll w/Beef & Rice	1 medium	6.0	2.7	26	2
Cannelloni, Meat & Cheese	1 piece	29.7	135.0	185	1
Cheese Souffle	1 cup	14.1	5.3	207	0
Chicken A La King, Hmde	1 cup	34.3	12.7	186	1
Chicken A La King w/Rice, Frzn	1 cup	12.0	4.0	122	1
Chicken & Dumplings	1 cup	10.5	2.7	103	1
Chicken & Rice Casserole	1 cup	18.0	5.1	103	1
Chicken & Veg. Stir-Fry	1 cup	6.9	1.2	26	3
Chicken Cacciatore, Frzn	12 oz.	11.0	3.8	80	1
Chicken Fricassee, Hmde	1 cup	18.1	5.2	85	1
Chicken-Fried Steak	4 oz.	23.4	6.8	115	0
Chicken Noodle Casserole	1 cup	10.7	3.2	59	2
Chicken Parmigiana, Hmde	7 oz.	17.0	5.9	150	2
Chicken Pot Pie	8 oz.	25.0	8.4	45	2
Chicken Salad, Regular	½ cup	21.2	9.1	56	0
Chicken Tetrazzini	1 cup	19.6	6.9	50	1
Chicken w/Cashews, Chinese	1 cup	28.6	4.9	60	2
Chili					
w/Beans Only	1 cup	12.0	4.0	35	7
w/Beans & Meat	1 cup	22.4	9.6	110	4

LUNCH/DINNER COMBOS (CONTINUED)

Item	Serving	Tot. Fat (g)	Sat. Fat (g)	Chol. (mg)	Fiber (g)
Chop Suey w/Rice Or Noodles	1 cup	10.5	3.6	50	2
Chow Mein, Chicken	1 cup	6.0	2.5	60	2
Corned-Beef Hash	1 cup	24.4	7.5	80	2
Crab Cake	1 small	4.5	0.9	90	0
Creamed Chipped Beef	1 cup	23.0	7.9	44	0
Deviled Crab	½ cup	15.4	4.1	50	1
Deviled Egg	1 large	5.3	1.2	109	0
Egg Foo Yung w/Sauce	1 piece	7.0	1.9	107	1
Eggplant Parmesan, Traditional	1 cup	24.0	8.7	31	3
Egg Roll	2	6.8	2.4	40	1
Enchilada					
Bean, Beef & Cheese	8 oz.	14.1	7.3	38	3
Beef, Frzn	8 oz.	16.0	8.7	40	2
Cheese, Frzn	8 oz.	26.3	14.7	61	3
Chicken, Frzn	8 oz.	16.1	6.4	65	4
Fajitas					
Chicken	1	15.3	3.0	41	4
Beef	1	18.2	6.1	34	3
Fettuccine Alfredo	1 cup	29.7	9.3	73	3
Fish And Chips, Frzn Dinner	6 oz.	14.8	4.3	25	3
Fish Creole	1 cup	5.4	0.9	60	2
Frozen Dinner					
Beef Tips And Noodles	12 oz.	15.1	6.2	75	4
Chopped Sirloin	12 oz.	30.1	14.3	130	5
Fried Chicken	12 oz.	29.6	7.4	110	6
Meat Loaf	12 oz.	23.1	6.4	65	4
Salisbury Steak	12 oz.	27.4	13.5	126	4
Turkey And Dressing	12 oz.	22.6	5.0	74	3
Green Pepper Stuffed w/ Rice & Beef	1 medium	13.5	5.8	52	2
Hamburger Rice Casserole	1 cup	21.0	7.7	57	3
Ham Salad w/Mayo	½ cup	20.2	4.4	54	0
Lasagna					
Cheese	8 oz.	12.0	4.8	22	3
w/Beef & Cheese	1 piece	19.8	10.0	81	2

Item	Serving	Tot. Fat (g)	Sat. Fat (g)	Chol. (mg)	Fiber (g)
Lobster					
Cantonese	1 cup	19.6	5.6	240	0
Newburg	½ cup	24.8	14.7	183	0
Salad	½ cup	7.0	1.5	36	0
Lo Mein, Chinese	1 cup	7.2	1.4	11	1
Macaroni & Cheese	1 cup	16.0	5.0	20	0
Manicotti, Cheese & Tomato	1 piece	11.8	6.0	61	2
Meatball (Reg. Ground Beef)	1 med	5.1	2.0	30	0
Meat Loaf w/Reg. Ground Beef	3 oz.	20.2	8.5	102	0
Moo Goo Gai Pan	1 cup	17.2	3.1	66	1
Moussaka	1 cup	8.9	2.8	98	3
Onion Rings	10 average	17.0	6.0	0	1
Oysters Rockefeller	6 oysters	12.5	4.0	70	1
Pepper Steak	1 cup	11.0	3.2	53	1
Pizza					
Cheese	1 slice	10.1	5.2	40	1
Cheese, French Bread, Frzn	5 oz.	13.0	6.7	37	1
Combination w/Meat	1 slice	17.5	9.0	56	1
Deep Dish, Cheese	1 slice	13.5	6.9	45	1
Pepperoni	1 slice	16.5	8.5	44	1
Tomato Only	1 slice	4.0	2.0	2	1
Pizza Rolls, Frzn	3 pieces	6.9	2.0	10	1
Pork, Sweet & Sour w/Rice	1 cup	7.5	2.0	31	1
Quiche					
Lorraine	⅛ pie	43.5	20.1	218	1
Plain Or Vegetable	1 slice	17.6	8.8	135	1
Ratatouille	½ cup	3.0	0.7	0	2
Ravioli, Canned	1 cup	7.3	3.6	20	3
Ravioli w/Meat & Tomato Sauce	1 piece	3.0	0.9	19	0
Sailsbury Steak w/Gravy	8 oz.	27.3	12.3	126	1
Salmon Patty, Traditional	4 oz.	12.5	4.1	94	1

LUNCH/DINNER COMBOS (CONTINUED)

Item	Serving	Tot. Fat (g)	Sat. Fat (g)	Chol. (mg)	Fiber (g)
Sandwiches (on whole wheat bread unless otherwise noted)					
BBQ Beef On Bun	1	16.8	5.8	54	4
BBQ Pork On Bun	1	12.2	3.7	56	4
BLT w/Mayo	1	15.6	4.1	23	4
Bologna & Cheese	1	22.5	9.7	42	4
Chicken w/Mayo And Lettuce	1	14.2	1.8	1191	4
Club w/Mayo	1	20.8	5.4	52	4
Corned Beef On Rye	1	10.8	3.2	34	4
Cream Cheese And Jelly	1	16.0	10.8	38	4
Egg Salad	1	12.5	2.5	228	4
French Dip, Au Jus	1	12.5	4.8	58	4
Grilled Cheese	1	24.0	12.4	56	4
Ham, Cheese & Mayo	1	16.0	7.3	29	4
Ham Salad w/Mayo	1	16.9	4.2	40	4
Peanut Butter & Jelly	1	15.1	2.3	10	5
Reuben	1	33.3	11.8	77	4
Roast Beef & Gravy	1	24.5	5.6	55	4
Roast Beef & Mayo	1	22.6	4.9	60	4
Sloppy Joe On Bun	1	16.8	5.8	54	4
Sub w/Salami & Cheese	1	41.3	17.7	109	4
Tuna Salad	1	17.5	2.9	17	4
Turkey & Mayo	1	18.4	1.9	17	4
Turkey Breast & Mustard	1	5.2	1.2	15	4
Shrimp Creole w/Rice	1 cup	6.1	1.2	123	2
Shrimp Salad	½ cup	9.5	1.6	69	1
Spaghetti					
w/Marinara Sauce	1 cup	2.5	1.0	5	2
w/Meat Sauce	1 cup	16.7	5.0	56	2
w/Red Clam Sauce	1 cup	7.3	1.0	17	2
w/Tomato Sauce	1 cup	1.5	0.4	5	2
w/White Clam Sauce	1 cup	19.5	2.6	49	1
Spaghettios	1 cup	2.0	0.5	8	2
Spinach Souffle	1 cup	14.8	7.1	184	2
Stroganoff					
Beef w/Noodles	1 cup	19.6	7.7	72	2
Beef w/o Noodles	1 cup	26.8	10.6	85	1

Item	Serving	Tot. Fat (g)	Sat. Fat (g)	Chol. (mg)	Fiber (g)
Sushi w/Fish & Vegetables	5 oz.	1.0	0.2	10	1
Taco, Beef	1 med	17.0	8.5	54	2
Tortellini, Meat Or Cheese	1 cup	15.4	5.4	238	1
Tostada w/Refried Beans	1 med	16.3	6.7	20	6
Tuna Noodle Casserole	1 cup	13.3	3.1	38	2
Tuna Salad					
Oil Pack w/Mayo	½ cup	16.3	2.7	20	0
Water Pack w/Mayo	½ cup	10.5	1.6	14	0
Veal Parmigiana	1 cup	22.5	10.1	75	0
Veal Scallopini	1 cup	20.4	7.3	132	2
Welsh Rarebit	1 cup	31.6	17.3	NA	0

MEATS (ALL COOKED W/O ADDED FAT UNLESS OTHERWISE NOTED)

Item	Serving	Tot. Fat (g)	Sat. Fat (g)	Chol. (mg)	Fiber (g)
Round, Eye Of, Lean	3 oz.	4.0	1.5	52	0
Beef, Lean, 5-10% Fat By Weight (Cooked)					
Flank Steak, Fat Trimmed	3 oz.	8.0	2.9	82	0
Hindshank, Lean	3 oz.	9.2	4.0	76	0
Porterhouse Steak, Lean	3 oz.	10.2	5.3	90	0
Rib Steak, Lean	3 oz.	9.2	5.0	80	0
Round Bottom, Lean	3 oz.	9.2	3.4	96	0
Roasted	3 oz.	7.2	2.7	81	0
Rump, Lean, Pot-Roasted	3 oz.	7.0	2.5	60	0
Top, Lean	3 oz.	6.2	2.2	89	0
Sirloin Steak, Lean	3 oz.	8.7	3.6	76	0
Sirloin Tip, Lean Roasted	3 oz.	9.2	3.9	90	0
Tenderloin, Lean, Broiled	3 oz.	11.0	4.2	83	0
Top Sirloin, Lean, Broiled	3 oz.	7.7	3.1	89	0
Beef, Regular 11-17.4% Fat By Weight (Cooked)					
Chuck, Separable Lean	3 oz.	15.0	6.2	105	0
Club Steak, Lean	3 oz.	12.7	6.1	90	0
Cubed Steak	3 oz.	15.2	3.3	85	0
Hamburger					
Extra Lean	3 oz.	13.9	6.3	82	0
Lean	3 oz.	15.7	7.2	78	0
Rib Roast, Lean	3 oz.	15.0	5.5	85	0
Sirloin Tips, Roasted	3 oz.	15.0	3.2	85	0

MEATS (CONTINUED)

Item	Serving	Tot. Fat (g)	Sat. Fat (g)	Chol. (mg)	Fiber (g)
Beef, Regular 11-17.4% Fat By Weight (Cooked) continued					
T-Bone, Lean Only	4 oz.	10.2	4.2	80	0
Tenderloin, Marbled	3 oz.	15.0	7.0	86	0
Beef, High Fat, 17.4-27.4% Fat By Weight (Cooked)					
Chuck, Ground	3 oz.	23.7	9.6	100	0
Hamburger, Regular	3 oz.	19.6	8.2	87	0
Meatballs	1 oz.	5.5	2.0	30	0
Porterhouse Steak, Lean & Marbled	3 oz.	19.5	8.2	80	0
Rib Steak	3 oz.	14.5	6.0	81	0
Rump, Pot-Roasted	3 oz.	19.5	8.2	80	0
Short Ribs, Lean	3 oz.	19.5	8.2	80	0
Sirloin, Broiled	3 oz.	18.5	7.7	78	0
Sirloin, Ground	3 oz.	26.5	9.3	84	0
T-Bone, Broiled	3 oz.	26.5	10.5	90	0
Beef, Highest Fat, = 27.5& Fat By Weight (Cooked)					
Brisket, Lean & Marbled	3 oz.	30.0	12.0	85	0
Chuck, Stew Meat	3 oz.	30.0	12.0	85	0
Corned, Medium Fat	3 oz.	30.0	14.9	75	0
Ribeye Steak, Marbled	3 oz.	38.6	12.0	90	0
Rib Roast	3 oz.	30.0	18.2	85	0
Short Ribs	3 oz.	31.5	10.5	90	0
Lamb					
Lean	3 oz.	8.0	3.4	100	0
Lean & Marbled	3 oz.	14.3	9.0	97	0
Loin Chop					
Lean	3 oz.	8.0	4.2	80	0
Lean & Marbled	3 oz.	22.3	11.7	58	0
Rib Chop					
Lean	3 oz.	8.0	5.0	50	0
Lean & Marbled	3 oz.	21.0	13.0	70	0
Liver					
Beef, Braised	3 oz.	4.8	1.9	400	0
Calf, Braised	3 oz.	6.8	2.3	450	0
Pork					
Bacon					
Cured, Broiled	1 strip	3.1	1.1	5	0

Item	Serving	Tot. Fat (g)	Sat. Fat (g)	Chol. (mg)	Fiber (g)
Pork (continued)					
Bacon (continued)					
Cured, Raw	1 oz.	16.3	6.0	19	0
Canadian Bacon, Broiled	1 oz.	1.8	0.6	14	0
Ham					
Cured, Canned	3 oz.	5.0	1.5	38	0
Cured, Shank, Lean	3 oz.	6.2	3.0	59	0
Marbled	2 slices	13.8	5.0	60	0
Fresh, Lean	3 oz.	6.3	1.5	40	0
Smoked	3 oz.	7.0	2.7	51	0
Smoked, 95% Lean	3 oz.	5.3	1.8	53	0
Loin Chop					
Lean	1 chop	7.7	3.0	55	0
Lean With Fat	1 chop	22.5	8.8	90	0
Rib Chop, Trimmed	3 oz.	9.8	3.5	81	0
Rib Roast, Trimmed	3 oz.	10.0	3.6	83	0
Sausage					
Brown And Serve	1 oz.	9.4	3.1	24	0
Patty	1	8.4	2.9	22	0
Regular Link	½ oz.	4.7	1.6	15	0
Sirloin, Lean, Roasted	3 oz.	10.0	3.6	85	0
Spareribs Roasted	6 med	35.0	11.8	121	0
Tenderloin, Lean, Roast	3 oz.	4.6	1.6	78	0
Top Loin Roast, Trimmed	3 oz.	7.5	2.8	77	0
Processed Meats					
Bacon Substitute (Breakfast Strips)	2 strips	4.8	1.0	0	0
Beef, Chipped	2 slices	1.1	0.4	15	0
Beef Breakfast Strips	2 strips	7.0	2.8	26	0
Beef Jerky	1 oz.	3.6	1.7	30	0
Bologna, Beef/Beef & Pork	2 oz.	16.2	6.9	33	0
Bratwurst					
Pork	2 oz link	22.0	7.9	51	0
Port & Beef	2 oz link	19.5	7.0	44	0
Chicken Roll	2 oz.	2.6	1.6	20	0
Corn Dog	1	20.0	8.4	37	0
Corned Beef, Jellied	1 oz.	2.9	1.0	3	0
Ham, Chopped	1 oz.	2.3	0.8	17	0

MEATS (CONTINUED)

Item	Serving	Tot. Fat (g)	Sat. Fat (g)	Chol. (mg)	Fiber (g)
Hot Dog/Frank					
Beef	1	13.2	8.8	27	0
Beef, Fat-Free	1	0.0	0.0	0	0
Chicken	1	8.8	2.5	45	0
97% Fat-Free Varieties	1	1.6	0.6	22	0
Turkey	1	8.1	2.7	39	0
Turkey, Fat-Free	1	0.0	0.0	0	0
Knockwurst/Knackwurst	2 oz link	18.9	3.2	36	0
Pepperoni	1 oz.	13.0	5.4	25	0
Salami					
Cooked	1 oz.	10.0	6.6	30	0
Dry/Hard	1 oz.	10.0	3.0	16	0
Sausage					
Italian	2 oz link	17.2	6.1	52	0
90% Fat-Free Varieties	2 oz.	4.6	1.6	40	0
Polish	2 oz link	16.2	5.8	40	0
Smoked	2 oz link	20.0	9.2	48	0
Vienna	1 sausage	4.0	1.5	8	0
Turkey Breast, Smoked	2 oz.	1.0	0.3	23	0
Turkey Ham	2 oz.	2.9	1.0	32	0
Turkey Loaf	2 oz.	1.0	0.3	23	0
Turkey Roll, Light Meat	2 oz.	4.1	1.2	24	0
Veal					
Blade					
Lean	3 oz.	8.6	3.5	100	0
Lean With Fat	3 oz.	16.5	7.0	100	0
Breast, Stewed	3 oz.	18.5	8.7	100	0
Chuck, Med. Fat, Braised	3 oz.	12.6	6.0	101	0
Cutlet Breaded	3½ oz.	15.0	NA	NA	0

NUTS AND SEEDS

Item	Serving	Tot. Fat (g)	Sat. Fat (g)	Chol. (mg)	Fiber (g)
Almonds	2 T	9.3	1.0	0	2.5
Brazil Nuts	2 T	11.5	2.3	0	2.5
Cashews, Roasted	2 T	7.8	1.3	0	2
Chestnuts, Fresh	2 T	0.8	0.0	0	4
Hazelnuts (Filberts)	2 T	10.6	1.0	0	2
Macadamia Nuts, Roasted	2 T	12.3	2.0	0	2.5
Mixed Nuts					
w/Peanuts	2 T	10.0	1.5	0	2
w/o Peanuts	2 T	10.1	2.0	0	2
Peanut Butter, Creamy	1 T	8.0	1.5	0	1
Peanut Butter, Chunky	1 T	8.5	2.5	0	2
Peanuts					
Chopped	2 T	8.9	1.0	0	2
Honey Roasted	2 T	8.9	1.5	0	2
In Shell	1 cup	17.0	2.2	0	4
Pecans	2 T	9.1	0.5	0	1
Pine Nuts (Pignolia)	2 T	9.1	1.5	0	2
Pistachios	2 T	7.7	0.8	0	2
Poppy Seeds	2 T	3.8	0.3	0	2
Pumpkin Seeds	2 T	7.9	3.0	0	2
Sesame Nut Mix	2 T	5.1	1.5	0	2
Sesame Seeds	2 T	8.8	1.2	0	2
Sunflower Seeds	2 T	8.9	1.0	0	2
Trail Mix w/Seeds, Nuts, Carob	2 T	5.1	0.9	0	3
Walnuts	2 T	7.7	0.3	0	2.5

PASTA, NOODLES AND RICE

Item	Serving	Tot. Fat (g)	Sat. Fat (g)	Chol. (mg)	Fiber (g)
Macaroni					
Semolina	1 cup	0.7	0.0	0	1
Whole Wheat	1 cup	2.0	0.4	0	3.5
Noodles					
Alfredo	1 cup	25.1	9.8	73	1
Angel Hair	1 cup	1.5	0.5	0	0
Cellophone, Fried	1 cup	4.2	0.6	0	0
Chow Mein	1 cup	8.0	1.6	0	0
Egg	1 cup	2.4	0.4	50	1
Fettucine, Spinach	1 cup	2.0	0.5	0	2
Manicotti	1 cup	1.0	0.2	0	1
Ramen, All Varieties	1 cup	8.0	5.0	0	1
Rice	1 cup	0.3	0.0	0	1
Romanoff	1 cup	18.0	11.9	95	3
Spaghetti, Whole Wheat	1 cup	1.5	0.5	0	3
Spaghetti, Enriched	1 cup	1.0	0.0	0	1
Rice					
Brown	½ cup	0.6	0.0	0	2
Fried	½ cup	7.2	0.7	0	2
Long Grain & Wild	½ cup	2.1	0.2	0	1
Pilaf	½ cup	7.0	0.6	0	1
Spanish Style	½ cup	2.1	1.0	0	0
White	½ cup	1.2	0.0	0	0

POULTRY

Item	Serving	Tot. Fat (g)	Sat. Fat (g)	Chol. (mg)	Fiber (g)
Chicken					
Breast					
w/Skin, Fried	½ breast	10.7	3.0	87	0
w/o Skin, Fried	½ breast	6.1	1.5	90	0
w/Skin, Roasted	½ breast	7.6	2.9	70	0
w/o Skin, Roasted	½ breast	3.1	1.0	80	0
Leg					
w/Skin, Fried	1 leg	8.7	4.4	99	0
w/Skin, Roasted	1 leg	4.8	4.2	85	0
w/o Skin, Roasted	1 leg	2.5	0.7	41	0
Thigh					
w/Skin, Fried	1 thigh	11.3	2.5	60	0
w/Skin, Roasted	1 thigh	9.6	2.7	58	0
w/o Skin, Roasted	1 thigh	4.5	2.4	45	0
Wing					
w/Skin, Fried	1 wing	9.1	1.9	26	0
w/Skin, Roasted	1 wing	6.6	1.9	29	0
Duck					
w/Skin, Roasted	3 oz.	28.7	9.7	84	0
w/o Skin, Roasted	3 oz.	11.0	4.2	89	0
Turkey Breast					
Barbecued	3 oz.	3.0	1.3	42	0
Honey Roasted	3 oz.	2.6	1.1	38	0
Oven Roasted	3 oz.	3.0	1.3	42	0
Smoked	3 oz.	3.3	1.4	49	0
Turkey Dark Meat					
w/Skin, Roasted	3 oz.	11.3	3.5	89	0
w/o Skin, Roasted	3 oz.	7.0	2.4	75	0
Ground	3 oz.	13.2	4.0	85	0
Ham	3 oz.	5.0	1.7	62	0
Turkey Light Meat					
w/Skin, Roasted	3 oz.	8.2	2.3	76	0
w/o Skin, Roasted	3 oz.	3.2	1.0	55	0
Roll, Light Meat	3 oz.	7.0	2.0	43	0
Sliced w/Gravy, Frzn	3 oz.	3.7	1.2	20	0

SALAD DRESSINGS

Item	Serving	Tot. Fat (g)	Sat. Fat (g)	Chol. (mg)	Fiber (g)
Blue Cheese					
Fat-Free	1 T	0.0	0.0	0	0
Low Cal	1 T	1.9	0.2	2	0
Regular	1 T	8.0	1.4	0	0
Buttermilk, From Mix	1 T	5.8	1.0	5	0
Caesar	1 T	7.0	0.9	13	0
French					
Fat-Free	1 T	0.0	0.0	0	0
Low Cal	1 T	0.9	0.1	1	0
Regular	1 T	6.4	0.8	0	0
Garlic, From Mix	1 T	9.2	1.4	0	0
Honey Mustard	1 T	6.6	1.0	0	0
Italian					
Creamy	1 T	5.5	1.6	0	0
Fat-Free	1 T	0.0	0.0	0	0
Low Cal	1 T	1.5	0.1	1	0
Item	Serving	Tot. Fat (g)	Sat. Fat (g)	Chol. (mg)	Fiber (g)
Oil & Vinegar	1 T	7.5	1.5	0	0
Ranch Style	1 T	6.0	0.8	4	0
Russian					
Low Cal	1 T	0.7	0.1	1	0
Regular	1 T	7.8	1.1	0	0
Thousand Island					
Fat-Free	1 T	0.0	0.0	0	0
Low Cal	1 T	1.6	0.2	2	0
Regular	1 T	5.6	0.9	0	0

SAUCES AND GRAVIES

Item	Serving	Tot. Fat (g)	Sat. Fat (g)	Chol. (mg)	Fiber (g)
Barbecue Sauce	1 T	0.3	0.0	0	0
Bearnaise Sauce, Mix	¼ cup	25.6	15.7	71	0
Beef Gravy, Canned	½ cup	2.8	1.3	4	0
Brown Gravy					
From Mix	½ cup	0.9	0.4	1	0
Hmde	¼ cup	14.0	6.5	5	0
Catsup, Tomato	1 T	0.1	0.0	0	0
Chicken Gravy					
Canned	½ cup	6.8	1.7	3	0
From Mix	½ cup	0.9	0.3	1	0
Giblet, Hmde	¼ cup	2.6	0.7	28	0
Chili Sauce	1 T	0.0	0.0	0	0
Cocktail Sauce	¼ cup	0.2	0.0	0	0
Guacamole Dip	1 oz.	4.0	0.7	0	0
Hollandaise Sauce	¼ cup	18.0	10.2	160	0
Home-Style Gravy, From Mix	¼ cup	0.5	0.2	0	0
Horseradish	¼ cup	0.1	0.0	0	0
Jalepeno Dip	1 oz.	1.1	0.4	60	0
Mushroom Gravy					
Canned	½ cup	3.2	0.5	0	1
From Mix	½ cup	0.4	0.2	0	1
Mustard					
Brown	1 T	1.8	0.3	0	1
Yellow	1 T	0.7	0.0	0	0
Onion Dip	2 T	6.0	3.7	13	0
Onion Gravy, From Mix	½ cup	0.4	0.2	0	0
Pesto Sauce	¼ cup	29.0	7.3	18	1
Picante Sauce	½ cup	0.8	0.1	0	2
Pork Gravy, From Mix	½ cup	1.0	0.4	1	0
Sour-Cream Sauce	¼ cup	7.6	4.0	28	0
Soy Sauce	1 T	0.0	0.0	0	0
Soy Sauce, Reduced Sodium	1 T	0.0	0.0	0	0
Spaghetti Sauce					
"Healthy"/"Lite" Varieties	½ cup	1.0	0.0	0	3
Hmde, w/Ground Beef	½ cup	8.3	2.3	23	2
Marinara	½ cup	4.7	0.7	0	3

SAUCES AND GRAVIES (CONTINUED)

Item	Serving	Tot. Fat (g)	Sat. Fat (g)	Chol. (mg)	Fiber (g)
Spaghetti Sauce (continued)					
Meat Flavor, Jar	½ cup	6.0	1.0	5	2
Mushroom, Jar	½ cup	2.0	0.3	0	2
Oil & Garlic	½ cup	4.5	1.5	5	0
Tomato	½ cup	2.2	0.5	0	0
Spinach Dip (sour-cream & mayo)	2 T	7.1	1.8	10	1
Steak Sauce					
A-1	1 T	0.0	0.0	0	0
Others	1 T	0.0	0.0	0	0
Tabasco Sauce	1 t	0.0	0.0	0	0
Tartar Sauce	1 T	8.2	1.5	0	0
Teriyaki Sauce	1 T	0.0	0.0	0	0
Turkey Gravy					
Canned	½ cup	2.4	0.7	3	0
From Mix	½ cup	0.9	0.3	1	0
Worcestershire Sauce	1 T	0.0	0.0	0	0

SOUPS

Item	Serving	Tot. Fat (g)	Sat. Fat (g)	Chol. (mg)	Fiber (g)
Asparagus					
Cream of, w/Milk	1 cup	8.2	2.1	10	1
Cream of, w/Water	1 cup	4.1	1.0	5	1
Bean					
w/Bacon	1 cup	5.9	6.0	3	4
w/Ham	1 cup	8.5	2.0	3	3
w/o Meat	1 cup	3.0	1.5	2	5
Beef, Canned					
Broth	1 cup	0.5	0.2	1	0
Chunky	1 cup	5.1	2.6	14	2
Beef Barley	1 cup	1.1	0.5	6	1
Beef Noodle Casserole	1 cup	3.1	1.2	5	1
Black Bean	1 cup	1.5	1.2	0	2
Broccoli, Creamy w/Water	1 cup	2.8	1.0	5	1
Canned Vegetable w/o Meat	1 cup	1.6	0.6	0	1

Item	Serving	Tot. Fat (g)	Sat. Fat (g)	Chol. (mg)	Fiber (g)
Chicken					
Chunky	1 cup	6.6	2.0	30	2
Cream of, w/Milk	1 cup	11.5	4.6	27	0
Cream of, w/Water	1 cup	7.4	2.1	10	0
Chicken & Dumplings	1 cup	5.5	1.3	34	0
Chicken & Stars	1 cup	1.8	0.7	5	1
Chicken & Wild Rice	1 cup	2.3	0.5	7	1
Chicken/Beef Noodle or Veg.	1 cup	3.1	1.2	5	1
Chicken Gumbo	1 cup	1.4	0.3	5	1
Chicken Mushroom	1 cup	9.2	2.4	10	1
Chunky Chicken Noodle	1 cup	5.2	1.1	18	2
Chicken Noodle w/Water	1 cup	2.5	0.7	7	0
Chunky Chicken Vegetable	1 cup	4.8	1.4	17	2
Chicken Veggie w/Water	1 cup	2.8	0.9	10	0
Chicken w/Noodles, Chunky	1 cup	5.0	1.4	19	2
Chunky Chicken w/ Rice	1 cup	3.2	1.0	20	2
Chicken Rice w/Water	1 cup	1.9	0.5	7	1
Clam Chowder					
Manhattan Chunky	1 cup	3.4	2.1	14	1
New England	1 cup	6.6	3.6	7	1
Consomme w/Gelatin	1 cup	0.0	0.0	0	0
Corn Chowder	1 cup	10.5	5.0	22	3.5
Crab	1 cup	1.5	0.4	10	0
Fish Chowder, w/Whole Milk	1 cup	13.5	5.3	37	1
Gazpacho	1 cup	1.5	0.5	0	3
Seafood Gumbo	1 cup	3.9	2.7	40	3
Lentil	1 cup	1.0	0.2	0	3
Lobster Bisque	1 cup	14.0	5.5	35	1
Minestrone					
Chunky	1 cup	2.8	1.5	5	2
w/Water	1 cup	2.5	0.8	3	1
Mushroom, Cream of					
Condensed	1 cup	23.1	10.1	30	1
w/Milk	1 cup	13.6	5.1	20	1
w/Water	1 cup	9.0	2.4	2	1
Mushroom Barley	1 cup	2.3	0.4	0	1
Mushroom w/Beef Stock	1 cup	4.0	1.6	7	1

SOUPS (CONTINUED)

Item	Serving	Tot. Fat (g)	Sat. Fat (g)	Chol. (mg)	Fiber (g)
Onion	1 cup	1.7	0.3	0	1
Onion, French w/Cheese	1 cup	7.5	2.5	15	0
Oyster Stew w/Water	1 cup	3.8	2.5	14	1
Oyster Stew w/Whole Milk	1 cup	17.7	2.5	14	0
Pea					
Split	1 cup	0.6	0.2	1	1
Split w/Ham	1 cup	4.4	1.8	8	1
Potato, Cream of w/Milk	1 cup	7.4	1.2	5	2
Tomato					
w/Milk	1 cup	6.0	2.9	17	1
w/Water	1 cup	1.9	0.4	0	0.5
Tomato Beef w/Noodle	1 cup	4.3	1.6	5	1
Tomato Rice	1 cup	2.7	0.5	2	1
Turkey Noodle	1 cup	2.0	0.6	5	1
Turkey Vegetable	1 cup	3.0	0.9	2	1
Vegetable, Chunky	1 cup	3.7	0.6	0	2
Vegetable w/Beef, Chunky	1 cup	3.0	1.3	8	2
Vegetable w/Beef Broth	1 cup	1.9	0.4	2	1
Vegetarian Vegetable	1 cup	1.2	0.3	0	1
Wonton	1 cup	1.0	<1.0	10	1

VEGETABLES

Item	Serving	Tot. Fat (g)	Sat. Fat (g)	Chol. (mg)	Fiber (g)
Alfalfa Sprouts, Raw	½ cup	0.1	0.0	0	0
Artichoke, Boiled	1 medium	0.2	0.0	0	3
Artichoke Hearts, Boiled	½ cup	0.1	0.0	0	3
Asparagus, Cooked	½ cup	0.3	0.1	0	2
Avocado	½ cup	25.0	4.0	0	3.5
Bamboo Shoots, Raw	½ cup	0.2	0.1	0	2
Beans					
All Types, Cooked w/o Fat	½ cup	0.4	0.2	0	9
Baked, Brown Sugar & Molasses	½ cup	1.5	0.2	0	4
Baked, Vegetarian	½ cup	0.6	0.3	0	5
Baked w/Pork & Tomato Sauce	½ cup	1.3	0.5	8	5

Item	Serving	Tot. Fat (g)	Sat. Fat (g)	Chol. (mg)	Fiber (g)
Beets, Pickled	½ cup	0.1	0.0	0	4
Broccoli					
Cooked	½ cup	0.3	0.0	0	7
Frzn, Chopped, Cooked	½ cup	0.1	0.0	0	2
Frzn In Butter Sauce	½ cup	1.5	1.0	<5	2
Raw	½ cup	0.2	0.0	0	1
Brussel Sprouts, Cooked	½ cup	0.4	0.0	0	2
Butter Beans, Canned	½ cup	0.4	0.0	0	4
Cabbage					
Chinese (Bok Choy)	1 cup	0.2	0.0	0	2
Green, Cooked	½ cup	0.1	0.0	0	2
Carrot					
Cooked	½ cup	0.1	0.0	0	2
Raw	1 large	0.1	0.0	0	2
Cauliflower					
Cooked	1 cup	0.2	0.0	0	3
Raw	1 cup	0.1	0.0	0	4
Celery					
Cooked	½ cup	0.1	0.0	0	1
Raw	1 stalk	0.1	0.0	0	1
Chinese-Style Vegetables, Frzn	½ cup	4.0	0.2	0	3
Chives, Raw, Chopped	1 T	0.0	0.0	0	0
Collard Green, Cooked	½ cup	0.1	0.0	0	2
Corn					
Corn On The Cob	1 medium	1.0	0.1	0	4
Cream Style, Canned	½ cup	0.5	0.1	0	4
Frzn, Cooked	½ cup	0.1	0.0	0	4
Cucumber					
w/Skin	½ medium	0.2	0.0	0	1
w/o Skin, Sliced	½ cup	0.1	0.0	0	0
Eggplant, Cooked	½ cup	0.1	0.0	0	2
Green Beans					
French Style, Cooked	½ cup	0.2	0.0	0	2
Snap, Cooked	½ cup	0.2	0.0	0	2
Italian-Style Vegetables, Frzn	½ cup	5.5	0.2	0	2
Kale, Cooked	½ cup	0.3	0.0	0	2

VEGETABLES (CONTINUED)

Item	Serving	Tot. Fat (g)	Sat. Fat (g)	Chol. (mg)	Fiber (g)
Kidney Beans, Red, Cooked	½ cup	0.5	0.0	0	8
Leeks, Chopped, Raw	½ cup	0.1	0.0	0	1
Lentils, Cooked	½ cup	0.4	0.0	0	8
Lettuce, Leaf	½ cup	0.2	0.0	0	1
Lima Beans, Cooked	½ cup	0.4	0.0	0	5
Mushrooms					
Canned	½ cup	0.2	0.0	0	1
Raw	½ cup	0.2	0.0	0	1
Mustard Greens, Cooked	½ cup	0.2	0.0	0	2
Okra, Cooked	½ cup	0.1	0.0	0	3
Olives					
Black	3 med	4.5	0.5	0	1
Greek	3 med	5.0	0.9	0	1
Green	3 med	2.5	0.2	0	1
Onions					
Canned, French Fried	1 oz.	15.0	6.9	0	0
Chopped, Raw	½ cup	0.1	0.0	0	1
Parsley, Chopped, Raw	¼ cup	0.1	0.0	0	0
Peas, Green, Cooked	½ cup	0.2	0.0	0	4
Pickles	1 medium	0.1	0.0	0	0
Pepper, Bell, Chopped, Raw	½ cup	0.1	0.0	0	2
Pimentos, Canned	1 oz.	0.0	0.0	0	0
Potato					
Baked w/Skin	1 medium	0.2	0.1	0	4
Boiled w/o Skin	½ cup	0.1	0.0	0	2
French Fries	½ cup	6.8	3.0	10	2
Hash Browns	½ cup	10.9	3.4	23	2
Mashed w/Milk	½ cup	5.0	1.5	5	1
Potato Pancakes	1 cake	12.6	3.4	93	1
Scalloped	½ cup	6.0	3.5	12	1
Pumpkin, Canned	½ cup	0.3	0.2	0	4
Radish, Raw	½ cup	0.2	0.0	0	1
Rhubarb, Raw	1 cup	0.2	0.0	0	2
Sauerkraut, Canned	½ cup	0.2	0.0	0	4
Scallions, Raw	½ cup	0.2	0.0	0	4
Soybeans, Mature, Cooked	½ cup	7.7	1.1	0	4

Item	Serving	Tot. Fat (g)	Sat. Fat (g)	Chol. (mg)	Fiber (g)
Spinach					
Cooked	½ cup	0.2	0.1	0	3
Creamed	½ cup	5.1	0.7	1	3
Raw	1 cup	0.2	0.0	0	3
Squash	½ cup	0.2	0.0	0	3
Succotash, Cooked	½ cup	0.8	0.1	0	3
Sweet Potato					
Baked	1 medium	0.2	0.0	0	6
Candied	½ cup	3.4	1.2	8	5
Tempeh (Soybean Product)	½ cup	6.4	0.9	0	1
Tofu (Soybean Curd), Raw	½ cup	5.4	0.8	0	1
Tomato					
Boiled	½ cup	0.5	0.0	0	1
Raw	1 medium	0.4	0.0	0	1
Stewed	½ cup	0.2	0.0	0	1
Turnip Greens, Cooked	½ cup	0.2	0.0	0	2
Wax Beans, Canned	½ cup	0.2	0.0	0	2
Yam, Boiled/Baked	½ cup	0.1	0.0	0	3
Zucchini, Cooked	½ cup	0.1	0.0	0	2

VARIOUS SNACKS

Item	Serving	Tot. Fat (g)	Sat. Fat (g)	Chol. (mg)	Fiber (g)
Cheese Puffs	1 oz.	10.0	4.8	14	0
Cheese Straws	4 pieces	7.2	6.4	5	1
Chex Snack Mix, Traditional	1 oz.	4.0	0.5	0	1
Corn Chips					
Barbecue	1 oz.	9.0	0.2	0	1
Regular	1 oz.	10.0	1.0	0	1
Cracker Jack	1 oz.	2.2	0.3	0	2
Mix (Cereal & Pretzels)	1 cup	2.5	0.5	0	2
Mix (Raisins & Nuts)	1 cup	25.0	3.5	1.5	4
Peanuts In Shell	1 cup	17.0	2.2	0	4
Popcorn					
Air Popped	1 cup	0.3	0.0	0	1
Caramel	1 cup	4.5	1.2	2	1
Microwave "Lite"	1 cup	1.0	0.0	0	1
Microwave, Plain	1 cup	3.0	0.7	0	1
Microwave, w/Butter	1 cup	4.5	1.8	1	1
Pork Rinds	1 oz.	9.3	3.7	24	0
Potato Chips					
Regular	1 oz.	11.2	2.9	0	1
Baked, Lays	1 oz.	1.5	0.0	0	2
Barbecue Flavor	1 oz.	9.5	2.6	0	1
Light, Pringles	1 oz.	8.0	2.0	0	0
Regular, Pringles	1 oz.	12.0	2.0	0	0
Pretzels (Hard)	1 oz.	1.5	0.5	0	1
Superpretzel® (Soft)	1 med.	1.0	0.0	0	2
Rice Cakes	1	0.0	0.0	0	0
Tortilla Chips					
Doritos	1 oz.	6.6	1.1	0	1
No Oil, Baked	1 oz.	1.5	1.0	0	1
Tostitos	1 oz.	7.8	1.1	0	1

Appendix
Famous Landmarks
and Walking Tours of
Philadelphia

"Philadelphia is the most walkable major city in the United States. As you stroll its streets, you'll be fascinated by the physical illustration of the progress of the centuries, the juxtapositions of past and present. Many neighborhoods are still made up of tree-lined, intimate streets flanked by lovely Federal town houses, especially in Society Hill, along Pine Street's Antique Row, and the residential streets west of Rittenhouse Square, such as Spruce, Locust, and Delancey. You'll notice the nearer you are to the Delaware River, the older (and smaller) the buildings are likely to be. The walking tours mapped out here are specifically designed to cover the most worthwhile attractions." (Lauren McCutcheon, "City Strolls" in *Frommer's Philadelphia and the Amish Country* 16th edition, Frommer's, May 2011.)

Some Major Attractions to Visit While Walking In Philadelphia:

City Hall

William Penn's 1683 plan for Philadelphia set Center Square, the largest of five, square-shaped "green-spaces" aside for the construction of public buildings. Until the late 19th century, Center Square was actually not the center of the city, as most of the population lived near the Delaware River and close to the Independence Hall.

As the population began to migrate westward, a need for a larger city hall was called for. Approved in 1870, Center Square was then renamed Penn Square in honor of the city's founder, William Penn.

Construction of the building began in 1871, designed by John McArthur, Jr. in the popular-for its day "Second Empire" style. While the project was to result in the "tallest building in the world," it was not completed until 1901 and had then been surpassed by the Eiffel Tower and the Washington Monument.

The central tower is 511 ft. tall. It is topped by a statue of William Penn. The giant statue is 37 ft. high and weighs 27 tons. It is just one of 250 sculptures created by Alexander Calder for both the interior and exterior of the building.

An observation deck is open to the public. City Hall Tour information and tickets are located in Room 121 at the East City Hall Entrance.

Society Hill

Bounded by Walnut, Lombard, Front and 8th streets and contains the largest concentration of original 18th and early 19th century architecture in the United States.

Society Hill's cobblestone streets are bordered by brick row houses that were built in the Federal and Georgian style.

Located close to both the Delaware River and Philadelphia's municipal buildings, such as Independence Hall, the neighborhood became the city's most populated area in which a number of 18th and 19th century market halls, taverns and churches were built and still exist today.

Other than Independence Hall, some significant Buildings to see in Society Hill are: The Society Hill Synagogue at 418 Spruce Street, erected in 1829 by Thomas U. Walter who was also one of the architects who designed the United States Capitol Building, The Oldest Independent African-American Church in the Nation, The Mother Bethel AME Church, located at 419 S. 6th St., and the Merchant's Exchange Building, built in 1832 by architect William Strickland and located at 143 S. 3rd Street.

Betsy Ross House

Built in 1740, Flag maker Betsy Ross rented this house located at 239 Arch Street in the Olde City section of Philadelphia from 1773 to 1786.

Mrs. Ross lived here with her husband, John, and the couple ran their upholstery business from the house.

Visitors take a tour that leads them through the cellar kitchen, the parlor, small bedrooms and living quarters, and also witness actors and actresses working on upholstery projects. The original upholstery shop is now a gift shop, where one can purchase flag-related mementos, books about Ross, and other colonial Philadelphia-related items.

The house is open 7 days a week, from Memorial Day until Labor Day. During the rest of the year, the house is open 6 days a week but is closed on Mondays. The Betsy Ross House is also closed on Thanksgiving, Christmas, and New Year's Day. Admission is free but a donation is suggested.

One Liberty Place

This symbolic skyscraper now synonymous with most popular images of Philadelphia's skyline became the first building to be built past the height of Philadelphia's City Hall. City Hall had been the tallest building in the city until 1987, when the construction of this new glass skyscraper far exceeding the city's central municipal building. Because an unwritten rule had been in existence prior to Liberty Place's construction preventing developers from building past the height of the hat on William Penn's statue atop the City Hall, the developer Willard G. Rouse had to change may minds in order to push the project through.

The first tower, One Liberty Place, was built in 1987. At 945 ft or 288 m it was the tallest building in the city until the completion of the Comcast Center in 2008. The postmodern 60-story tower, with a blue glass exterior, was designed by Murphy & Jahn Associates.

In 1990 a smaller but related tower, two Liberty Place, was built adjacent to the first building. Liberty Place is located in Center City, at 17th and Chestnut Streets.

The Museum of Art

The Philadelphia Museum of Art is one of the country's largest art museums. Its collection holds more than 300,000 works of art including photographs, paintings, tapestry, carpets, sculpture, armory, ceramics and furniture. Within its 200 galleries there are reconstructed Buddhist and Hindu Temples, a Chinese Scholars' study and a Japanese Tea Garden. Its paintings collection includes works from renowned artists like Picasso, Van Gogh, Rubens and Renoir, and from local and national artists such as Charles Wilson Peale and Thomas Eakins.

The Museum is located on a hill at the end of the Benjamin Franklin Parkway, providing a perfect vista for this wide boulevard and also to the majestic Schuylkill River and Boathouse Row at its back.

In 1907 the decision was made to build this new museum on a hill known as Faire Mount, at the end of the recently completed Benjamin Franklin Parkway. The building, designed by Horace Trumbauer, Julian Abele, Clark Zantzinger and Charles Borie, was inspired by the design of Greek temples such as the Parthenon.

Benjamin Franklin Parkway

In 1891, a proposal was submitted to the Philadelphia city council to create a wide road connecting City Hall with the city's largest green space, Fairmount Park. In 1907 an updated plan designed by Paul Crét and Horace Trumbauer was approved and the buildings lining the area were torn down to make way for the new boulevard. Modeled in part after the Champs-Elysees in Paris, a final set of plans by Jaques Greber and Cret for the parkways' creation was submitted and accepted in 1917 by the Fairmount Park Commission.

Logan Square is the central point on the Parkway, and now goes by the name of Logan Circle. Originally one of the "five squares" in William Penn's original plan for Philadelphia, it was redesigned by Gréber as a large traffic circle similar to the Place de la Concorde. At the center is a large fountain, the Swann Memorial Fountain. It was built in 1924, two years before the official completion of the Benjamin Franklin Parkway.

A great number of religious, cultural, and educational institutions are clustered along the parkway. Among them are the Franklin Institute, the Academy of Natural Sciences, the Free Library of Philadelphia, the Cathedral of Sts. Peter and Paul, the Rodin Museum, and the Museum of Art, which provides an amazing anchor to the end of the Parkway.

Rittenhouse Square

Rittenhouse Square was originally called Southwest Square due to its location in that part of the city. Like the other squares drawn up by William Penn, it was not only meant as a "green space" for the city's citizens to mingle but was also a site where livestock roamed about. In 1816, the residents who lived next to or near the square asked that it be enclosed by a fence and raised funds to do so. In the next several decades, trees and walkways were added as were the first houses facing the square. The name of Southwest Square was changed in 1825 to honor David Rittenhouse, a Philadelphia astronomer and instrument maker.

By the late 19th century, Rittenhouse Square was noted by many commentators as the place where Philadelphia's Victorian aristocracy lived, and some of their homes remain on the streets of the square today.

A number of distinctive sculpture have been placed here since the mid to late 19th century, including the 1832 "Lion Crushing a Serpent" by French Romantic sculptor Antoine-Louis Barye and "Duck Girl of 1911" by Paul Manship.

Elfreth's Alley

Located in the Olde City section of the city, the alley is known as the nation's oldest continually occupied street. Established in 1702, most of the homes that still remain were built between 1728 and 1836, and an estimated 3,000 people have lived there throughout the centuries.

Throughout much of the 18th and 19th centuries, artisans and craftsmen lived in the houses that lined the alley and often ran businesses out of their homes. Much later, during the Industrial Revolution, many of those same houses in the Alley became home to European immigrants.

At 126 Elfreth's Alley, you can visit the Elfreth's Alley Museum, which was originally built and owned by the alley's namesake, the Blacksmith Jeremiah Elfreth. A guided tour of the home is an option but visitors can also tour on their own as well.

Fairmount Park Water Works

Philadelphia's first water works was planned as a response to the Yellow Fever epidemic of 1793. Forming a "watering committee" in 1799, the city adopted a design by Benjamin Latrobe, who proposed a steam engine system to do the job but soon after was replaced by John David and Frederick Graff's new design in 1812. Comprising a 3 million gallon reservoir and a pump house using steam engines to pump water, a

1,600-foot dam was also built across the Schuylkill which moved water to three wooden wheels, replacing Latrobe's steam engine.

As the first large-scale municipal water works in the nation, the site was nationally and internationally lauded, and was the model for similar facilities throughout the U.S and abroad. With its Greek Revival architectural style and its appealing waterside location, the water works often attracted many visitors each year, and even Charles Dickens stated of the site that it was "no less ornamental than useful, being tastefully laid out as a public garden."

While the original Fairmount Water Works finally closed its doors in 1909, today it has been renovated and turned into an interpretive history center and is also a National Historic Landmark.

Christ Church Burial Ground

Among the most famous of the many Philadelphians interred here include 5 signers of the Declaration of Independence, including Benjamin Franklin.

Franklin, who died in 1790, is buried alongside his wife Deborah and children Francis and Sarah. Franklin's grave is visible day and night through a metal fence without actually having to set foot in the cemetery. The burial ground is open daily and public or private tours are available.

Other early Americans and signers of the Declaration buried at Christ Church include Francis Hopkinson, Joseph Hewes, Dr. Benjamin Rush, and George Ross.

And, also buried in Christ Church cemetery are heroes from the Revolutionary War and World War I, as well as several Pennsylvania and United States Government officials, authors and poets, others.

Independence Mall

The term "Independence Mall" was a moniker given to this historic district in 1945, when a large area north of Independence Hall was designated as Independence Mall State Park. In 1946, Pennsylvania Governor Ed Martin provided the required funding to create the Independence Mall. The money was necessary because of the need to purchase and subsequently demolish buildings covering nearly nine city blocks in order to design a large enough space to lead up to both the historic 18th century building and to its adjacent historic sites.

Construction began in 1951 but would not be finished until 1967. The National Park Service took over the administration of the site in 1973, and the Independence Mall became a part of the larger Independence National Historical Park. Today, Independence Mall has the feel of a large urban park, surrounded by a number of historic buildings, such as the Liberty Bell Pavilion and the National Constitution Center. The Mall is often a hot-spot for musical performances, food-festivals and a number of events that are typically sponsored by the city of Philadelphia.

Boathouse Row

Located between Kelly Drive and the Schuylkill River, the Victorian houses of Boathouse Row all have their own unique history. Visible from the city's Schuylkill Expressway, these houses are home to the oldest amateur athletic governing body in America and have been on the National Register of Historic Places since 1987.

Much of Fairmount Park's rowing activities come out of these 12 houses. Ten of them belong to rowing clubs, including those of Philadelphia's Big 5 Universities—Penn (University of Pennsylvania), Temple, St. Joseph's, Villanova, and La Salle.

These rowing clubs were organized in the mid to late 19th century, and their boat houses were generally built between the 1870s and the early 1900s. The Bachelors Barge Club is the oldest continuously operating rowing club in America, and was started by a group of volunteer firefighters who were stationed near the river.

The houses of Boathouse Row are beautiful during the day, but viewing them at night is perhaps even more memorable as tens of thousands of lights light up their facades along the Schuylkill River.

Reading Terminal Market

In the early days of colonial America, outdoor "farm" markets were quite popular. They provided fresh, local foods for people who lived in cities such as Philadelphia and were often conveniently located in the centers of towns.

As these markets decreased in number by the late 19th century, the city of Philadelphia in a partnership with the Reading Railroad opened the Reading Terminal Market in 1892.

The building that housed the original market and still does today was designed by F. H. Kimbal, and at the time of its erection was one of the largest single-span arched roof structures in the world.

When it opened, the Reading Terminal Market, located below the railroad terminal itself, had room for up to 800 vendors. Eventually, they would set up shop in small, six-foot stalls, including many Amish vendors from Southeastern and Central Pennsylvania.

The Reading Terminal Market eventually closed in 1976 but a revitalization campaign brought the Market back to its old position of prominence and today the Market is an amazing place for locals and visitors to enjoy lunch or shop for fresh seafood, meat, veggies, fruit, and desserts to take home for dinner. There are also numerous vendors selling books, clothing, and arts and crafts.

The Italian Market

Located in South Philadelphia, the Italian Market is situated along eight to ten blocks of Ninth Street, is one of the largest open-air markets in America and has been in continual operation since the late 19th Century. Originally organized and operated by Italian immigrants who resided in the neighborhood, it now includes food and crafts from a variety of Italian, Southeast Asian, and Mexican traditions, reflecting the new diversity of ethnicities living in the area. You can find almost anything at the market, as vendors sell fresh fruits and vegetables, as well as meats, fish, and spices. Coffee shops restaurants and other gourmet establishments also line the blocks, including butcher shops and bakeries. More specifically, there are a number of Mexican taquerias along with several bodegas, Southeastern Asian and Vietnamese cuisine shops like pho soup and banh mi (Vietnamese hoagie shops), and many Italian restaurants can also be found in the market. And of course, Philly Cheesesteaks from Philadelphia's famous cheesesteak stands are located in the Italian Market.

BIBLIOGRAPHY

Edward Colimore, *The Philadelphia Inquirer's Walking Tour of Historic Philadelphia* (Philadelphia Inquirer's Walking Tours of Historic Philadelphia) Camino Books, (February 28, 2007)

Streetwise Maps, Streetwise Philadelphia Map—Laminated City Center Street Map of Philadelphia, PA—Folding pocket size travel map with Septa metro map, bus map Streetwise Maps (September 1, 2011)

Doug Gelbert, *A Walking Tour of Philadelphia—Old City, Pennsylvania* (Look Up, America!) [Kindle Edition] Cruden Bay Books (May 23, 2009)

Roslyn F. Brenner *Philadelphia's Outdoor Art: A Walking Tour* Camino Books; 2nd edition (May 2002)

Lauren McCutcheon and Carrie Havranek, *Frommer's Philadelphia and the Amish Country* (Frommer's Complete Guides) Frommers; 16th edition (May 31, 2011)

John Gattuso, *Insight City Guide: Philadelphia. Long Island City*: Langenscheidt Publishers, 2007.

Richard Varr, *Eyewitness Travel: Philadelphia and the Pennsylvania Dutch Country.* New York: DK Publishing, Inc., 2007

Walking Tour Websites:

http://www.theconstitutional.com/

http://www.visitphilly.com/tours/walking-tours/

http://www.nationalgeographic.com/walkingtours/Philadelphia_Walking_Tour/index.html

http://preservationalliance.com/events/walking_tours.php

http://www.ghosttour.com/philadelphia

http://www.frommers.com/destinations/philadelphia/0023010008.html

SUBJECT INDEX

T

U

V

W

Y